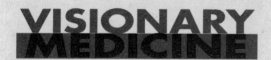

VISIONARY MEDICINE
REAL HOPE FOR TOTAL HEALING

By Simone Gabbay

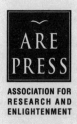

ARE
PRESS

ASSOCIATION FOR
RESEARCH AND
ENLIGHTENMENT

A.R.E. Press • Virginia Beach • Virginia

A.R.E. Press
215 67th Street
Virginia Beach, VA 23451-2061

Library of Congress Cataloguing-in-Publication Data
Gabbay, Simone, 1956–
    Visionary medicine : real hope for total healing / by Simone Gabbay.
        p.   cm.
Includes index.
    ISBN 0-87604-472-0 (trade paper)
    1. Holistic medicine. 2. Cayce, Edgar, 1877–1945–Contributions in holistic medicine. I. Title.
R733.G325 2003
613–dc21

2002156490

A Note to the Reader:
No part of this book is intended to substitute for competent medical diagnosis, nor does the A.R.E. endorse any of the information contained herein as prescription for the treatment of disease. Edgar Cayce gave health readings for particular individuals with specific conditions; therefore, any application of his advice in present–day treatment planning should be undertaken only after consulting with a professional practitioner in a related field. It is especially important that you do not discontinue any prescribed treatment without the full concurrence of your doctor.

Cover design by Richard Boyle

Dedication

To my beloved mother, the late Helga Seefeldt,
whose physical and emotional hurts
first prompted me to study and research
the Edgar Cayce readings, and who,
though we had differing philosophies,
first taught me about the power of prayer
and the healing power of love.

She crossed over just before I completed this book.

Contents

Acknowledgments

I offer my gratitude to God and His Holy Spirit for giving me the opportunity, the strength, and the ability to write this book. Working on this project was my response to a calling I heard several years earlier, and I feel blessed to have been an instrument of God in its manifestation.

Thanks to the wonderful people who have given their support to this project:

- Dr. John O.A. Pagano, who took the time to review the entire manuscript and offer helpful suggestions and expertise. Dr. John, you were an answer to prayer!
- Ken Skidmore, my brilliant editor at A.R.E. Press, who patiently worked with me on the fine points of the manuscript and never grew tired of my revisions and additions. Ken, we were meant to work together on this project, and I'm grateful that we succeeded in the second round!
- Dr. Dudley Delany, who has been an untiring supporter of my work and who kindly contributed the section on The Radial Appliance and Wet Cell Battery in chapter 6. Dudley, you are a true friend in Christ!
- Francis Sporer, who provided his knowledge and expertise of the Cayce/Reilly massage. Francis, you could have written this book better than I, and I greatly appreciate your help!
- My husband, Eliahu, and our son, Benjamin, who encouraged me throughout the joys and pains of writing this book and never complained about the many evening and weekend hours that I spent at the computer. I thank you both for your precious love and support!

I would also like to thank my friends and associates who, in many ways, have encouraged and inspired me in my work on this book: Jay D. Allen, Alice Bonnefoi, Rev. David Alan Bruce, Aranka de Szegheo, Moreah Ragusa Fach, Susan A. Lendvay, Andrea Lemieux, Catherine MacDonald and James Schmidt, Ruben E. Miller, Dr. William A. McGarey, T. Kay Rix, Jon and Robin Robertson, Dr. Lance H.K. Secretan, Monieca Seddon, A. Robert Smith, Sandra Tonn, and Frank and Nancy Thomas. Last but not least, a special thank you to Cathy Merchand at A.R.E. Press.

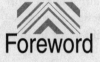

Foreword

SIMONE GABBAY HAS done it again! Following on the heels of her outstanding book *Nourishing the Body Temple* (1999, A.R.E. Press), *Visionary Medicine: Real Hope for Total Healing* correlates the health information made available to us by the Edgar Cayce readings with modern scientific data as does no other book in existence today. Ms. Gabbay's style of writing makes "easy reading" out of information generally thought to be beyond the scope of the lay reader, demonstrating her thorough knowledge of the subject. This was made evident to me by the mere fact that I could not put the book down once I began reading it! The late Gina Cerminara, Ph.D., author of several books on Cayce, said it most succinctly: "The secret of good writing is to be understood," to which I would like to add "with no chance of being misunderstood." Ms. Gabbay's writing is a perfect example of that principle in action.

More than just an array of Cayce readings and documented scientific findings, this book sheds light on some of mankind's most dreaded diseases, suggesting approaches that have not even been considered in the past. In its accuracy and thoroughness it offers hope where, heretofore, there was none. Perhaps most important of all, it reinforces the movement toward the amalgamation of holistic healing and modern medicine. It informs the scientific community, as well as suffering humanity, that when all else fails, don't despair, there just may be another way. Only a closed mind would not be moved by the vast wealth of information this book offers with reference points all along the way.

Visionary Medicine: Real Hope for Total Healing carries us through ancient as well as modern concepts of healing, riding high on the crest of a wave into the future. It reviews where we were, reveals where we are, and projects where we are going. It is not a book to be put on a book shelf and forgotten. It is to be placed on your night stand, on your kitchen counter, or on the coffee table in your living room, for immediate and constant accessibility. It is a compilation of health material for the lay person as well as for physicians and health practitioners of every kind that promises to be a guiding light on the subject of healing now and for many years to come.

Dr. John O. A. Pagano, Chiropractic Physician
Author of *Healing Psoriasis: The Natural Alternative*
January 20, 2003

Introduction

THE MAN WHO has been called the father of the holistic health movement never went to medical school. Although he was not a physician, his advice brought help and healing to the thousands of individuals who consulted him for various conditions, ranging from headaches and influenza to stomach ulcers, leukemia, and multiple sclerosis. Even today, more than half a century after his death, Edgar Cayce's recommendations are being studied and successfully applied by health care professionals and lay persons, who continue to find an inexhaustible resource in the more than fourteen thousand psychically channeled discourses that he provided during his lifetime. Approximately two-thirds of these discourses, referred to as readings, were related to questions of physical health. However, in true holistic fashion, the readings always addressed the involvement of mind and spirit in physical conditions, emphasizing that healing could not occur unless body, mind, and spirit were harmonized and brought into balance.

Edgar Cayce was a remarkable diagnostician, who, in his self-induced hypnotic state, was able to telepathically "scan" another person's body and accurately determine its condition, along with symptoms and their causes, and to recommend therapies and remedies that would help to correct the ailment. Tapping into what the readings said was a pool of universal consciousness, Edgar Cayce was able to bypass the guessing stages of medical diagnosis and aim straight at the root cause of a pathological condition, while simultaneously designing a unique course of treatment that was most likely to benefit the person for whom help was being sought. It didn't matter whether that person was in the same room with Cayce or going about his or her activities in another town or country. Cayce was able to access the information pertaining to that individual with the same speed and apparent ease. However, the energy required to enter into and maintain an altered state of consciousness each time he gave a reading was considerable, and his health suffered as a result.

It was a price that Edgar Cayce, who was born in 1877 near Hopkinsville, Kentucky, willingly paid for the fulfillment of his ardent desire to be helpful to others. He had nurtured this wish from a very young age. He felt drawn to Christian ministry, and although his family's circumstances did not allow him to pursue the theological studies he aspired to, his extensive knowledge of the Bible, which he read from cover to cover once for every year of his life, paved the way for him to teach Sunday School. However, it was ultimately through his psychic readings that his prayers for a missionary life were answered on a scale much larger than he had imagined, for the spiritual wisdom contained in these readings continues to inspire and help people all over the world.

Even as a young boy, Edgar Cayce displayed special gifts and had the ability to communicate with those who had passed on. His favorite playmates were other-dimensional beings, such as elves and fairies. In school, the young Edgar had difficulty following the curriculum until he discovered that he was able to sleep on a book and remember its entire contents upon awakening. This helped his grades to improve dramatically. It was not until he reached his early twenties, however, that his remarkable powers became apparent. He had developed a condition known as *aphonia*, marked by the loss of his voice. There was no known cure, and Cayce and his family had almost resigned themselves to the idea that he would have to live with this problem for the rest of his life. When offered the opportunity to consult a hypnotist, Edgar Cayce agreed to try a session, thinking that he had nothing to lose. During the experiment, while in a hypnotic state, Cayce spoke in a normal voice, accurately diagnosing the cause of his psychosomatic condition as nervous tension. He went on to recommend that he be given the hypnotic suggestion to increase circulation to the affected area, which would serve to normalize the condition. Miraculously, the suggestion worked, and Cayce regained the use of his voice.

Impressed with the remarkable results of the experiment, the hypnotist, who was also a student of osteopathy and a self-taught practitioner of suggestive therapeutics, encouraged Cayce to try out his newly discovered diagnostic powers on some of his clients who had failed to receive help from conventional medical doctors. In the ensuing experiments, the readings consistently proved accurate and helpful when the often unusual course of treatment they suggested was followed. The therapies and remedies that were prescribed in the readings appeared to incorporate the wisdom and knowledge of several different schools of healing. From diet and massage to herbal remedies and unique electromechanical appliances designed to regulate body energies, the recommendations did not appear to favor any particular discipline. However, they were often unorthodox and always aimed at balancing body, mind, and spirit to bring about complete and lasting healing.

No one was more surprised by the information that presented itself through him than Cayce himself. In his normal waking state, he had only a very basic understanding of anatomy and was unfamiliar with much of the medical terminology that formed part of the readings' vocabulary. Some of the medicaments and remedies mentioned were so unusual that even seasoned health professionals had never heard of them, yet they were ultimately found to exist and be effective.

For many years, Cayce refused to accept compensation for his readings, not wanting to use for personal gain a gift he had received from God. He provided a modest living for himself and his family through his work as a professional photographer. Eventually, however, the growing number of requests for readings forced him to dedicate himself to this calling on a full-time basis. When he died in 1945, Edgar Cayce left the rich legacy of his readings, which had been stenographically re-corded by his devoted secretary, Gladys Davis. Now fully catalogued and available on CD-ROM, the readings are accessible for study through the Association for Research and Enlightenment (A.R.E.) in Virginia Beach, Virginia, where Cayce and his family had settled in 1925. It was there that in 1929, backed by a group of supporters, Cayce realized his dream of establishing a hospital where the treatments recommended in the readings could be administered to patients. Although financial dif-ficulties forced the hospital to close in 1931, the building is today once again part of the work begun by Cayce. It houses several of the A.R.E.'s management offices, as well as its Health and Rejuvenation Center, which offers Cayce-style treatments to the public, and the Cayce/Reilly School of Massotherapy, which provides professional training for mas-sage therapists and offers a variety of holistic studies.

Dr. Harold J. Reilly, the founder of the school, was a physiotherapist, chiropractor, and naturopath. Although he and Edgar Cayce had never heard of each other, Reilly was singled out in the readings as the health professional best able to carry out many of the prescribed treatments. In 1930, when patients started coming to his practice in New York with referrals from Edgar Cayce, Reilly was surprised to find that the diag-noses and treatment recommendations the patients brought with them originated in psychic readings. The material presented by the patients seemed plausible enough, however, for the open-minded Reilly to carry out Cayce's instructions. Encouraged by the positive results of the treat-ments, Reilly became fascinated with the phenomenon of the psychic diagnostician and began a lifelong study of the readings. After the clo-sure of his famous Reilly Health Institute in Rockefeller Center in 1965, Harold Reilly set up a physiotherapy clinic in Virginia Beach—the fore-runner of today's Health and Rejuvenation Center.

Dr. Reilly's name became synonymous with the concept of Cayce-style therapeutic massage, hydrotherapy, and exercise. Even today, years after his death in 1987 at the age of 92, Reilly's best-selling book, *The Edgar Cayce Handbook for Health Through Drugless Therapies*, continues to edu-cate its readers in the practical knowledge of Cayce's health programs, medically tested by the health professional who was specially chosen in the readings.

While the original Cayce hospital survived only two years from 1929 to 1931, Edgar Cayce's dream of a health establishment where the treatments conceived in the readings could be administered was again realized when the A.R.E. Clinic in Phoenix, Arizona, opened in 1970. Since its inception, thousands of patients have been treated there under the leadership and guidance of Dr. William A. McGarey, an internationally acclaimed physician and author of several books on the Cayce material.

Having researched and professionally applied the medical information in the Cayce readings for over forty years, McGarey remains one of the outstanding pioneers who have worked tirelessly to educate both health care professionals and lay persons about the importance of integrating body, mind, and spirit in all efforts to bring about healing. It is largely due to the unique combination of medical expertise and spiritual insight with which McGarey has approached this task that the Cayce therapies have become firmly established in the early history of modern holistic healing.

Today, many independent health professionals around the world continue to research and apply the suggestions from the Cayce readings. Dr. John O.A. Pagano, a chiropractic physician and author of the best-selling *Healing Psoriasis: The Natural Alternative* and *Dr. John's Healing Psoriasis Cookbook,* has had outstanding successes in curing many of the most stubborn cases of psoriasis with treatment methods that are based on the recommendations of Edgar Cayce. A look at the before-and-after photographs of some of Dr. Pagano's patients whose severely cracked and irritated skin became lesion-free within months of following the suggested treatment provides a glimpse of the enormous healing potential that such natural methods have.

Dr. Dudley Delany, a now retired chiropractor, massage therapist, and registered nurse, used the Cayce-recommended Radial Appliance, the Wet Cell Battery, and other suggestions from the readings to overcome multiple sclerosis, a disease considered to be incurable by mainstream medicine. Delany's inspiring book *The Edgar Cayce Way of Overcoming Multiple Sclerosis: Vibratory Medicine* is a fountain of hope for the estimated two and a half million people worldwide who suffer from this often debilitating condition.

Since 1989, in-depth research into the health information from the

Edgar Cayce readings has been undertaken in an organized manner through Meridian Institute in Virginia Beach, an independent nonprofit organization created with the goal to research holistic and integrative approaches to wellness and healing. Meridian Institute is working to establish protocols for the treatment of specific diseases based on the Edgar Cayce health readings. Its work is helping to promote the integration of mainstream medicine with alternative medicine and holistic modalities.

Today, more than half a century after Edgar Cayce's death, the health information from the Cayce readings remains at the cutting edge of modern holistic medicine—waiting to be explored, applied, and fully understood as the concepts of spirituality, psychoneuroimmunology, and mind–body healing are being validated by mainstream medical research.

Holistic Medicine: An Integrative Approach to Healing Body, Mind, and Spirit

All healing is one, whether in the laying on of hands, by word of mouth, by mechanotherapy, mechanical applications or what not. God is the Creative Force that gives life—and not the medicine or the application!

Edgar Cayce reading 1663-1

A QUIET REVOLUTION is underway in health care. The standard medical system of diagnosing and treating illness has become increasingly complex and technology-oriented, and many informed consumers are turning toward alternative methods of healing. A growing discontent with orthodox allopathic medicine's heavy reliance on drugs and surgery has prompted patients to seek out gentler, less intrusive methods of treatment. This subtle, yet very noticeable shift in the direction of alternative therapies signals a renewed appreciation of an ancient omnipresent source of health: the *vis medicatrix naturae*, as the healing power of nature is referred to in naturopathic medicine.

For thousands of years, people all over the world have relied on traditional healing methods, many of which are rooted in the understanding that the cause of illness lies in a violation of the laws of nature, and that only a full realignment with these laws can achieve a complete and lasting cure. The specific ways in which these natural laws are understood differ from culture to culture, but individually each approach can be viewed as one of several possible interpretations within the multidimensional complexity of nature. As such, no system is totally right or wrong, but each forms an integral part of a larger picture. Metaphorically understood, healing within nature might be seen as a hologram wherein each method, while being an essential part of the whole, is also fully capable of initiating complete healing in and of itself.

The holistic approach to medicine, which incorporates both the wisdom of ancient healing traditions and the more recently developed modalities of naturopathy and other therapeutic techniques, is based on this all-encompassing concept of healing. The word "holistic" is derived from the Greek *holos*, which translates into "whole" or "complete." Holistic healing, therefore, acknowledges the essential unity of body, mind, and spirit, as well as the interconnectedness between an individual's state of health and his or her environment. The natural therapies employed in a holistic system of healing are tailored to the unique needs of the individual and aim to correct specific imbalances that have resulted in the manifestation of *dis-ease* and less-than-perfect health.

For instance, a holistic practitioner's "prescription" for a patient suffering from severe migraine headaches might include a detoxification program, dietary changes, therapeutic massage and spinal manipulation, homeopathic remedies or flower essences, and stress management training. Each of these therapies, and others not specified here, are likely to be helpful when used alone, but the synergistic effect of several appropriate modalities employed together will significantly speed up the healing process and serve to increase the patient's awareness of the many factors that play a role in producing or alleviating symptoms of physical discomfort and illness.

Compared with the standard allopathic approach to treating migraines, which would typically offer a prescription for potent painkillers, the holistic course of treatment appears at first more d. follow. It requires considerable commitment on the part of the and it frequently demands a significant lifestyle change. The long-term benefits, however, are well worth these efforts, since the patient will ultimately not only be relieved of the migraine headaches, but will also enjoy generally improved health and increased physical and mental well-being, free of the unpleasant side effects usually associated with a drug-based approach.

Despite its strong emphasis on natural methods, the holistic philosophy of healing acknowledges that pharmaceutical drugs and surgery may be appropriate when used in the acute stages of illness and are helpful tools that often save lives when an injury or accident have occurred. The holistic approach views the relationship between allopathic and alternative medicine as complementary rather than antagonistic, and it welcomes the opportunity of cooperation. Thus, any method that helps to stimulate the body's own healing energies is a welcome tool for the holistic practitioner, who knows that all healing comes from one source, as Cayce reading 969-1 explains: "... *from whence comes the healing? Whether there is administered a drug, a correcting or an adjustment of a subluxation, or the alleviating of a strain upon the muscles, or the revivifying through electrical forces; they are* one *and the healing comes from* within."

The role of the holistic medical practitioner, then, is to help create the correct environment and the appropriate external conditions that will facilitate the awakening of the body's innate healing energies, whether this is done through conventional or alternative therapies.

In Europe, where natural health care practices such as homeopathy, hydrotherapy, and therapeutic massage already form an integral part of the mainstream medical system, patients enjoy a wide range of alternative treatment options. Allopathic and alternative therapies exist side by side and are frequently used in combination by medical practitioners in private practice and in clinical settings. When there's an emphasis on cooperation rather than mistrust, the patient benefits. Ralph Moss, Ph.D., an internationally respected researcher of alternative cancer therapies, writes in the February/March 2001 issue of the *Townsend Letter for Doctors and Patients* about the integration of conventional and alternative cancer therapy in European clinics: "In all, I think that the treatments offered at these German, Swiss and Scandinavian clinics represents [sic] the best hope for cancer patients. They do not reject the good parts of conventional oncology, but attempt to integrate that knowledge into a more humane and rational treatment philosophy."

In North America, the process of integrating alternative therapies into mainstream medicine is considerably slower. Cancer patients looking for alternative methods of treatment are often forced to leave the country if they want to find a clinic that offers natural therapies. However, it is estimated that 80 percent of cancer patients in the United States use special diets, nutritional supplements, and herbal remedies in addition to conventional treatment.

In their search for healing of everyday aches and pains, too, Americans are embracing alternative therapies with great enthusiasm: A national survey published in the November 11, 1998, issue of the *Journal of the American Medical Association* showed that the number of Americans using alternative therapies rose from about 33 percent in 1990 to more than 42 percent in 1997. A smaller survey conducted by a private-sector company in March 2000 indicated that nine out of ten Americans believe that alternative medicine may help to heal a wide range of health conditions. The most popular forms of alternative therapies used were supplements of vitamins and herbs, followed by massage, aromatherapy, yoga, and homeopathy.

Nearly half of all asthma and seasonal allergy sufferers also seek relief by using alternative therapies, according to a survey conducted by medical staff at the University of California, San Francisco, in 2001. And a surprising report published in the December 2001 issue of the *Journal of the American Geriatrics Society* showed that 30 percent of Americans age sixty-five and older use at least one alternative therapy—most commonly herbs, chiropractic, vitamin supplements, relaxation techniques, and religious healing.

Even the government is listening: in March 2000, responding to a growing demand for natural therapies by the American public, President Clinton issued an executive order to establish a White House Commission on Complementary and Alternative Medicine Policy, designed to coordinate research and increase knowledge about complementary and alternative practices and products. In the same year, the National

Center for Complementary and Alternative Medicine, a part of the National Institutes of Health (NIH), made public a new database of literature on complementary and alternative medicine through the Internet, accessible at www.nccam.nih.gov. This database allows members of the public to access a large number of abstracts, references, and some full-text articles on alternative medicine. With more than one hundred million Americans regularly using the Internet to find information on health topics, this type of reference tool will go a long way toward helping both health care givers and consumers to educate themselves about alternative therapies.

Perhaps this new Internet tool will also encourage much-needed communication about such therapies between physicians and patients. Studies have shown that when patients use alternative medicine, they seldom tell their allopathic physicians. Whether they fear that their doctor would advise them to discontinue the alternative therapies, or whether they feel that there's no need for the doctor to know, many who use vitamins, herbs, or guided imagery and meditation don't volunteer this information to their medical care givers, according to a study done with cancer patients at the University of Pennsylvania in 2000. This means that many patients who take prescription drugs are also taking herbal remedies or dietary supplements without their doctor's knowledge, potentially exposing themselves to the risk of drug/supplement interactions. Research on such interactions only began recently and is still in its very early stages.

We do know, however, that pharmaceutical drugs can have harmful side effects all on their own. The extent of the damage done by these known side effects is far more serious than the chance that someone will be hurt, or even die, as a result of taking a herbal or dietary supplement. A close-up look at the long list of casualties from pharmaceutical drug and hospital errors can help shed light on this issue.

Dangers of Pharmaceutical Drugs

When you think of the side effects of pharmaceutical drugs, what comes to mind? Headaches, fatigue, dizziness? Though they are unpleasant, these symptoms appear harmless when compared to a far more serious side effect: death. The results of a study published in the *Journal of the American Medical Association* in April 1998 indicate that adverse drug reactions are a major cause of death among hospitalized patients. What is particularly disturbing is that these reactions occur despite the fact that the drugs are administered correctly.

According to a November 1999 report released by the Institute of Medicine (IOM), more than 7,000 people are estimated to die annually in the U.S. due to medication errors. As many as 98,000 patients die as a result of medical errors in hospitals each year. In the U.K., a report issued by the Audit Commission in 2001 says that the number of Britons dying in hospital from medication errors and the adverse effects of medicines rose dramatically from 200 in 1990 to 1,100 in 2000. The report states that complications arising from medication are the most common cause of adverse events in hospital patients.

In March 2000, the diabetes drug trogliatazone (Rezulin) was withdrawn from the market following a request from the U.S. Food and Drug Administration (FDA). The drug, designed to lower blood sugar in diabetics, had been linked to sixty-three deaths and ninety confirmed cases of liver failure. The following year, the cholesterol drug Baycol was pulled from the market by its manufacturer, Bayer AG, following thirty-one deaths in the U.S. from a muscle-related side effect. In early 2002, this number was revised upward to about one hundred known deaths.

Serious side effects, including nerve damage and death, have also been observed in patients taking the arthritis drugs Enbrel and Remicade. In 2001, the FDA issued recommendations to physicians advising that patients who develop neurological symptoms after taking Enbrel or Remicade should discontinue the drug immediately. Another arthritis drug, Arava, has been implicated in severe liver reactions, some with fatal outcomes, according to a statement issued by the European Medicines Evaluation Agency (EMEA) in March 2001.

Even if they don't lead to death, the side effects of pharmaceutical drugs can be highly debilitating. A report in the January 2002 issue of *Neurology* points out that common drugs that act on the brain chemical serotonin, including some antidepressants, decongestants, and migraine medications, may trigger a stroke in rare cases. And results of a study released by researchers from Ohio State University in 2001 indicate that chemotherapy administered to women with breast cancer causes rapid bone loss in women, thus increasing the risk of osteoporosis. Bone–thinning was also observed in patients over the age of 60 who had taken corticosteroids for longer than six months, according to a report in the October 23, 2000, issue of the *Archives of Internal Medicine*. Corticos–teroids are prescribed for chronic inflammatory conditions, including rheumatoid arthritis and multiple sclerosis.

Other research suggests that some medications may prolong or worsen the conditions that they are intended to relieve. Doctors at the University of Maryland found that flu sufferers who took one of the antifever medications such as aspirin and acetaminophen were sick an average of 3.5 days longer than people who did not take these drugs. Alternative practitioners who work with natural methods will not be surprised by these findings because they know that a fever is nature's effective mechanism that allows the body to rid itself of pathogens and toxins, and that when fevers are suppressed, the toxic condition in the body will persist.

In other research, the migraine–fighting drug Maxalt–MLT was shown to worsen headaches in patients sensitive to aspartame, an artificial sweetener that is added to the drug, which is designed to melt on the tongue rather than being swallowed. In addition to triggering head–aches, Aspartame has been associated with a multitude of side effects, including glandular imbalances, joint pains, vomiting, memory loss, vision problems, and miscarriage.

Despite the high number of medication–related deaths each year, and despite the multiple side effects being reported, doctors and patients appear to hold on to their faith in the effectiveness of prescription drugs. U.S. physicians issued 9 percent more prescriptions for pharmaceuticals in 1999 than in the previous year, with each doctor writing an average of 2,060 prescriptions. According to a study conducted at the University of Medicine and Dentistry of New Jersey in New Brunswick, the major–ity of these prescriptions were not called for and were written in re–sponse to patient requests or subtle pressuring of doctors by patients. Perhaps if doctors and patients had greater awareness of the many un–desirable side effects of pharmaceutical drugs, doctors would exercise more caution when prescribing them, and patients would not be as eager to leave their physician's office with a prescription.

One example of drugs that are frequently overprescribed is antibiotic medication. According to a survey conducted by researchers at Massachusetts General Hospital in Boston, out of 2,000 trips to doctors' offices during the ten-year period from 1989 to 1999, 73 percent of patients who visited their doctor complaining of a sore throat received a prescription for antibiotic drugs, even though most sore throats are caused by viruses, which do not respond to antibiotics. In the decade covered by the survey, prescriptions of the macrolide antibiotics for children rose by a staggering 320 percent.

According to the American College of Physicians–American Society of Internal Medicine (ACP–ASIM), antibiotic treatment of colds, bronchitis, and other upper-respiratory infections is "almost always inappropriate," and these conditions are better treated with over-the-counter cold remedies and old-fashioned home remedies, such as saltwater gargles.

Over-prescribing antibiotics increases the chances that bacteria will become resistant to these drugs, a phenomenon that is already occurring at an alarming rate with strep infections and pneumonia-fighting drugs. This trend is particularly disturbing because it lowers the overall effectiveness of antibiotic medication for serious and life-threatening conditions—the only justifiable and appropriate use of antibiotics. The problem of drug resistance has become so severe that in September 2001, the World Health Organization launched a global initiative to stem the spread of bacteria that are resistant to antibiotics.

But there is more at stake than increased drug resistance. Antibiotics wipe out the healthy microflora in the intestinal tract, which is essential for the proper synthesis and absorption of nutrients in the small intestine. Such a disruption in the intestinal microflora causes various vitamin and mineral deficiencies. It also suppresses the immune system and frequently contributes to an overgrowth of undesirable yeast organisms, such as *Candida albicans*. Numerous health problems, including chronic fatigue, multiple food allergies, and hyperactivity in children, have been linked to yeast overgrowth in the intestines. Physicians prescribing antibiotics, and patients taking them, should be aware that in order to keep *Candida* in check, and to promote a healthy intestinal environment, it is important to take a probiotic supplement containing both *Lactobacillus acidophilus* and *Bifidobacterium bifidum* following a course of antibiotics.

The insidious dangers of the excessive use of antibiotics for both humans and animals became apparent in early January 2002, when meat from livestock fed with animal feed tainted with a powerful antibiotic that can stop blood cell production was feared to have reached supermarket shelves in several European countries. This is one of the most serious examples of drug abuse and one of the most insidious ways in which drug resistance is unintentionally promoted. By routinely administering antibiotics to humans and animals, we run the risk of sabotaging one of the most effective and potentially helpful medical discoveries of our time.

Prescription drugs load the body with toxins. They deplete nutrients, disrupt metabolism, and have the potential to cause addiction. The health problems caused by these side effects are often "treated" with yet more drugs, setting the stage for multiple chemical dependencies. Children as young as age three are put on this roller coaster with behavior-modifying drugs such as Ritalin and Prozac, which is now marketed in a mint-flavored liquid, easily administered to those too young to swallow tablets. Sadly, they are also too young to recognize that they are being infused with a potentially dangerous psychiatric drug. Research done at the University of Buffalo found that Ritalin, a drug frequently prescribed for children diagnosed with hyperactivity or attention-deficit disorder, may cause long-term changes in the brain. It's too bad that most pediatricians don't seem to know that hyperactivity often ceases on its own when refined and processed foods are eliminated from children's diets.

Unfortunately, things don't seem to be getting better for our kids. A survey conducted by Medco Health in 2002 revealed that prescription drug use among children is rising at an unprecedented rate. According to the survey, spending on prescription drugs for infants, children, adolescents, and young adults had increased 85 percent during the previous five years, making this group the fastest-growing prescription users in 2001.

The elderly, too, are at special risk of developing health problems related to the side effects from medication. In fact, drug reactions are frequently the reason why elderly patients end up in the emergency department at hospitals, according to a report published in the December 2001 *Annals of Emergency Medicine*. With many older people taking several prescription drugs every day, reactions are often aggravated by the interaction of two or more such drugs. Some drugs can even interfere with or cancel the effects of other drugs. For instance, acetaminophen can increase the anticlotting effect that another drug, warfarin, has in the blood, thus raising the risk of bleeding.

Pharmaceutical drugs are chemicals which are unnatural to the body. They acidify the system, thus contributing to lymphatic congestion. The lymphatic system, which is the body's major waste removal mechanism, needs an alkaline environment for optimal function. Drugs also burden the liver, which is responsible for detoxifying the body from the fallout of chemical substances. Most drugs also rob the body of B vitamins, especially folic acid. Calcium and potassium are depleted by antacids, antifungal drugs, and anti-inflammatory medication (corticosteroids). The resulting nutritional imbalances can cause wide-ranging digestive and metabolic problems.

Prescription drugs can and do save lives. Sometimes they are necessary. But in many cases, a dietary change, a herbal extract, or a nutritional supplement, along with a change in lifestyle, can provide the body with the necessary elements to promote healing at a fraction of the cost, and without causing further damage. These are the gentler, safer "prescriptions" that are provided under a holistic naturopathic treatment program.

The High Cost of Unnecessary Medical Procedures

Decades ago, the late Robert S. Mendelsohn, M.D., an internationally renowned pediatrician and author of several books on health, including *Confessions of a Medical Heretic*, wrote: "I don't advise anyone who has no symptoms to go to the doctor for a physical examination. For people *with* symptoms, it's not such a good idea, either . . . You should be aware of the dangers, and that even the simplest, seemingly innocuous elements can be a threat to your health and well-being."

Dr. Mendelsohn believed that many medical tests and procedures caused more harm than good, and today, a growing number of physicians and health advisors would agree with him. Common tests such as EKGs, angiograms, biopsies, mammograms, and Pap tests, all have critics who contend that the tests either fail to detect when there is a problem, creating a false sense of security, or that inaccurate results from these tests often encourage the use of expensive and invasive medical procedures that are unnecessary and of questionable benefit to the patient.

According to research published in the November 20, 2001, issue of the prestigious British medical journal *The Lancet*, the Ayre's spatula, a tool commonly used by doctors for Pap smears, is "an ineffective device." And experts from the Centers for Disease Control and Prevention in Atlanta, Georgia, write about the Pap smear in the November 10, 2001, issue of the *Morbidity and Mortality Weekly Report*: "Women who were screened annually rather than less frequently might have worse health outcomes if low-grade results of undetermined clinical importance lead to further testing and unnecessary patient morbidity and anxiety."

Results of a national survey released by the Robert Wood Johnson Foundation in May 2001 show that the vast majority of doctors and nurses say they have personally witnessed a "serious" medical mistake, and that fundamental changes to the American health care system are required to improve the quality of care. Medical mistakes range from the misdiagnosis of the cause of a cough or sore throat (doctors accurately determine whether coughs or sore throats are caused by a bacterium or a virus in only 50 percent of cases) to the deaths from prescription drugs mentioned earlier.

In an effort to reduce the incidence of medical errors in hospitals, the U.S. Department of Health and Human Services (HHS) is considering to propose regulation that would require drug manufacturers to put bar codes on their products. These bar codes could then be compared to bar codes that hospital patients would have on their identification bracelet, thus helping to avoid incidents where patients are given the wrong medication or wrong dosages of medication. In Italy in January 2002, the Health Ministry launched an Internet-based network program that will monitor drug reactions by inviting physicians to submit reports of adverse effects from drugs after they have been placed on the market. It is hoped that this "pharmacovigilance" network will help to prevent deaths and serious complications from adverse drug reactions.

In the meantime, our high–technology oriented, drug–based health care system is costing us not only lives and health, but also lots of money: By spring 2001, employer health premiums had risen 11 percent over the previous year, up from 8 percent in 2000, and 5 percent in 1999. But all our expensive drugs and medical procedures don't seem to be able to make us healthier. Cardiovascular disease remains the leading cause of death in the United States. It afflicts a staggering 61,800,000 Americans, according to a report released by the American Heart Association (AHA) in December 2001. In 1999, deaths from cardiovascular disease totaled nearly one million, and accounted for 40 percent of all deaths during that year. Cardiovascular disease includes such conditions as high blood pressure, stroke, heart attack, chest pain, and congestive heart failure. The AHA report points out that the cost of caring for patients suffering from cardiovascular disease amounts to billions of dollars each year and will continue to escalate.

Another factor that drives up health care costs is obesity. Worldwide, the number of overweight people is estimated at 1.2 billion. The United States has the highest percentage of obese (excessively fat) people in the world, with about 20 to 30 percent of all adults falling in the obese range. Obesity accounts for up to 7 percent of health care costs in the U.S., compared to only 2 percent in France and Australia. An illness that is directly related to poor diet and physical inactivity, obesity is implicated in as many as 300,000 deaths each year in the U.S. Those who are obese are also at increased risk of many other diseases, including diabetes, stroke, arthritis, depression, and several forms of cancer.

Diet and lifestyle also play an important role in the development of type 2 diabetes, which is 90 percent preventable, according to a report in the September 13, 2001, issue of *The New England Journal of Medicine*. An estimated sixteen million Americans have type 2 diabetes, a condition in which the body is unable to properly use the hormone insulin, which controls blood sugar and regulates its absorption for cellular energy. Diabetics, in turn, are at increased risk of other debilitating conditions such as coronary heart disease, kidney damage, nerve degeneration, and impaired or lost vision and hearing.

Many of the conditions that dramatically drive up health care costs—including heart disease, obesity, and diabetes—are known to be preventable. It should alarm us that billions of dollars are being spent on prescription drugs and on complicated medical tests and procedures in a failing attempt to control health problems that directly result from poor diet, unhealthy lifestyle, and lack of exercise. To help heal these conditions, we don't need more money for drug research. We only need to return to more natural ways of living and eating—the very principles upon which holistic medicine is built.

The Mind-Body Connection

One aspect of healing that allopathic medicine had neglected far too long is the concept that the mind plays an important role in creating health or illness in the body. A steady stream of medical research papers now confirms what many traditional systems of healing and the Edgar Cayce readings have consistently emphasized: An individual's state of mind has a direct influence on the body's health and well-being. The Cayce readings point out the importance of holding the right mental attitude: *"What aids [the] body? . . . The keeping of the mental attitude that is ever constructive . . . "* (641–6) and *" . . . a great many of the angles or attitudes in the physical forces of the body are brought about by the mental attitude that is held—and through same make for those building influences in the body."* (270–34)

"The placebo effect," in which the belief in the effectiveness of a medication can of itself produce the effect even though the medication is inactive, was found to be real and measurable in a study done at the University of British Columbia in Vancouver, Canada. In the study, Parkinson's disease patients who took an inactive placebo drug experienced a substantial increase in the release of the brain chemical dopamine. In individuals suffering from Parkinson's, the release of dopamine is impaired. Although the authors of the study call for further research into the question of placebos, the implications of their findings are truly phenomenal, providing a glimpse into the power of the mind to influence physical processes.

In another study, an individual's state of mind was found to directly influence whether and to what extent they experienced lower back pain. Researchers at the Stanford University Medical Center in California found that those who suffered from depression or had poor coping skills perceived lower back pain as more seriously debilitating than those who did not allow themselves to become discouraged by the thought of a physical problem, such as a torn disk, in the lower vertebrae.

The mind's reaction to stress can also lead to illness. A study reported in the July 2001 issue of *Hypertension: Journal of the American Heart Association* revealed that the perception of high job strain was associated with higher diastolic blood pressure in study subjects. In an earlier study from Finland, men who had a high degree of hopelessness in their lives were found to be three times as likely to develop high blood pressure than those with a positive outlook on life. The Cayce readings frequently encourage us to keep up hope: "Do *keep sweet. Keep that attitude of expectancy. Do keep the attitude of hope. And* know *that there is healing in the power and might of the love of God."* (2948-1)

Indeed, the belief in God itself appears to have a positive influence on health and longevity, according to a report published in the journal *Health Psychology* in 2000. Those who regularly attended a church, synagogue, mosque, or Buddhist monastery had a reduced risk of health problems, such as high blood pressure or heart disease and lower mortality and increased survival rates than those who did not. In several other studies, prayer and meditation were found to help lower blood pressure and reduce the risk of heart disease. Clearly, a mind that is focused on God is good for the health of the body.

The mind may even be as powerful as being able to hold off death. According to a study reported in the April 4, 2001, issue of *The Journal of the American Medical Association*, a conspicuously high death rate in at least one hospital in the month of January 2000 points to the possibility that some individuals may have willed themselves to stay alive through the Y2K period, in order to witness the much-publicized occasion.

When we engage the power of the mind in any effort to produce healing of the body, we greatly increase our chances of success. According to the Cayce readings, it is helpful to " . . . *[keep] all well under the influence of the mental forces of self, knowing that all healing properties must come from within, and as the mental holds the relation to self, and to the I AM within, just so will the response of each applied force from without respond from within."* (42–1)

The readings offer many suggestions for how we can help ourselves to better health by using natural therapies and remedies. In subsequent chapters of this book, we will explore some of these suggestions, along with the parallels that exist in traditional and modern modalities of holistic healing.

Holistic Nutrition:
Let Food Be Your Medicine

... while spiritual thought and spiritual food values are essentially supplying elements to a physical body, in the material plane it is necessary also that material food values be taken for sustaining not only the physical forces but the spiritual elements as well; to keep them in contact or as parallel one to another in their activity. Edgar Cayce reading 516-4

DIET AND HEALTH are inextricably connected. The foods we ingest are broken down in digestion and then used as building blocks for the cells that make up the body. It stands to reason, then, that the quality of the building blocks has a direct effect on the strength and integrity of the body cells into which they are assimilated. Weak cells are prone to disease and degeneration, while strong cells can ward off illness and promote good health and longevity. Every day, new research is published that tells us about the benefits of a natural whole foods diet for cellular health, and the damage done by refined, processed foods.

Yet, diet is one of the most neglected aspects of health. Pressed by chronic lack of time and the hectic pace prevalent in our modern world, we feel that we have no choice but to eat fast—to eat on the run and hope that the body will manage, at least for now, with fast-food snacks and store-bought dinners delivered from freezer to dinner table in less than ten minutes by the magic of the microwave oven. After all, if we'd take an hour to prepare and eat dinner, we wouldn't be able to go to our fitness class!

We buy "healthy" snacks and dinners, to be sure, preferably those labeled low-fat, calorie-reduced, and cholesterol-free! But we've been misled by claims that these are health foods. And our bodies are the (barely) living proof: obesity, heart disease, and diabetes are rampant and are fast approaching epidemic levels in the industrialized world.

We recognize that education is the key to reversing this trend, and so we've started to teach school children about good nutrition. We tell them what foods are good to eat, but we blindly repeat the concepts with which mainstream nutrition, influenced by powerful food-processing conglomerates, has been inoculating the media-mind: Eat a variety of foods from the four food groups, but choose low-fat, calorie-reduced, and cholesterol-free foods. Never mind if these foods are processed and refined, chemically altered, or loaded with additives and preservatives. Eat these things and you'll grow strong and healthy!

To make matters worse, we teach the children nothing about the importance of chewing foods well and slowly, and that the attitude with which the food is prepared and eaten influences its health-giving properties. In school, we rush the kids through lunch and snack breaks, paving the path for a lifelong habit of gulping food down quickly and inattentively. And then we wonder why the incidence of obesity and degenerative disease is increasing even among children.

So, despite hundreds of nutrition titles appearing on bookstore shelves each year and numerous magazine articles competing for the quickest-yet-nutritious ten-minute weeknight dinners, perhaps it's time to admit to ourselves that we still haven't quite got it—we still don't know how to eat well and keep ourselves healthy. Perhaps it's time to take another look at diet—not only at the types of foods we should or shouldn't eat, but also at the way in which they are prepared and, especially, at the way in which they are eaten.

The Cayce readings on diet leave no doubt that food is considered to be of primary importance in the effort to build a healthy body. In fact, the contribution made by food is said to be one of the two most important health–building tools in reading 288-38: " . . . *what we think and what we eat—combined together—*make *what we* are; *physically and mentally."*

A profound statement with far–reaching implications that mirrors a concept often emphasized in the readings: that the food we eat affects both the health of the body and the health of the mind and that the thoughts we think do the same thing. One of the pioneers who have established evidence for the way in which nutrition affects the mind is Dr. Abram Hoffer, an orthomolecular psychiatrist, who has found that blood sugar imbalances are implicated in 60 percent of schizophrenia cases, and that mild cases of the illness respond well to treatment with high doses of niacin, a member of the B complex of vitamins. B vitamins are known to play an important role in preserving the health of the nervous system. Recent studies have also shown that the adequate intake of another member of this group of vitamins, folic acid, decreases the risk of developing Alzheimer's disease.

Research published in the December 2001 issue of the *European Journal of Clinical Nutrition* indicates that a healthy diet may indeed protect the elderly against mental decline. The authors of the study, Dr. M.L. Correa Leite and colleagues from the National Research Council in Milan, Italy, suggest that antioxidants such as vitamins C and E may be key nutrients in this process. Antioxidants, which are compounds that mop up damaging free radicals in the body, have been shown to protect against degenerative conditions, including heart disease and some types of cancers.

Even a teenager's mental health is benefited by good dietary habits, especially if they include regular family meals, according to a study published in the February 2002 issue of the *Journal of Epidemiology and Community Health*. The results of this study showed that those teens who shared the least meals with their family were seeking mental health care more frequently than their peers who dined in the company of other family members on a more frequent basis. This research points not only to the importance of eating regular meals, but also to the more intangible aspects of nutrition, namely the fact that the environment and ambience in which the meals are taken has a direct influence on how the body receives and assimilates its nourishment. As Cayce said in reading 900–393, " . . . *the body should eat—and should eat slowly; yet when worried, overtaxed, or when the body may not make a* business *of the eating, but eating to pass away the time, or just to fill up time, not good—for it* will not *digest . . .* "

Indeed, we need to learn how to make a proper business of eating. It's one of the most important things we can do for our health.

Building Immunity with Vegetables and Fruit

The historical Greek physician Hippocrates said, "Let your food be your medicine and your medicine your food . . . There is a healing power inherent in nature." More than two millennia later, scientific research is substantiating Hippocrates' statement, as well as the dietary guidelines from the Cayce readings, with a flood of studies confirming the powerful influence that diet has on the body.

A study in 1997, supported by the National Heart, Lung, and Blood Institute, identified a diet that appears to help prevent heart disease, cancer, high blood pressure, and diabetes. Such a diet consists of fresh vegetables and fruit, with proportionately smaller amounts of whole grains, natural dairy products, naturally raised meat, poultry, and fish, as well as dried beans, nuts, and seeds. These recommendations are surprisingly similar to those that were given in the Edgar Cayce readings more than fifty years earlier. The readings emphasize the importance of a diet that is 80 percent alkaline forming, meaning that this portion of the diet should consist of fruits and vegetables, which are the foods that, after being metabolized, leave alkaline–forming mineral elements in the body. Meats, grains, and most fats and dairy products, on the other hand, produce an acid residue.

The key issue is that optimal metabolic function depends on the proper acid–alkaline balance, or pH balance, of body fluids. Most body fluids must be kept slightly alkaline, and a diet high in fruits and vegetables contributes to this alkalinity. The Cayce readings repeatedly stress the fact that a predominantly alkaline diet supports immune function and helps to prevent the common cold and influenza. Reading 1947–4 states: *"Keep the body alkaline! Cold germs do not live in an alkaline system! They do breed in any acid or excess of acids of any character left in the system."*

Through their alkalizing properties, fruits and vegetables also protect against bone loss by preventing an over-acidity in the body. Consuming large amounts of meat and starches produces an acid condition for which the body tries to compensate by pulling calcium—an alkaline-forming mineral—into the bloodstream. By increasing fruit and vegetable intake, this process can be both prevented and reversed.

Fresh fruits and vegetables not only contribute to alkalinity in the body—they also provide an abundance of vitamins and minerals that are equally important in maintaining proper immune function. Researchers at Pennsylvania State University, whose study showed that a healthy diet may indeed support the immune system and keep it youthful, even into old age, believe that the vitamins and minerals supplied by such a diet are key elements in preserving immune system health.

Other studies have shown that a diet high in vegetables can help to protect against two major killer diseases: cancer and diabetes. In particular, colon and lung cancer occur less frequently in those who eat lots of veggies. Lycopene, a micronutrient abundantly supplied by ripe tomatoes, has been shown to protect against certain types of cancer, including cancer of the prostate. The bioavailability of lycopene is higher in cooked and processed tomatoes, especially in tomato sauce. It is interesting to note that the Cayce readings, which recommend plenty of raw foods in general, state that canned tomatoes—preserved without chemicals—are preferable to raw tomatoes that are not fully vine-ripened. Vine-ripened fresh tomatoes are generally only available during a few short weeks in late summer. A good rule of thumb, therefore, is to eat fresh and raw tomatoes when they are in season, and to use lycopene-rich cooked and naturally preserved tomatoes at other times.

Eating vegetables also helps to normalize high blood pressure, a condition that up to 90 percent of middle-aged and older Americans can expect to experience at some point during their lives. In a study by Duke University Medical Center, a group of patients with high blood pressure was put on a diet high in fresh fruits and vegetables. After only two weeks, the average blood pressure dropped to levels previously attainable only with medication. It is interesting to note that this group had a near-normal salt intake, yet most high blood pressure patients are told by their doctors to eliminate or severely reduce sodium consumption. This study shows, however, that adding a few servings of vegetables to the daily diet achieves better results than tossing out the salt shaker!

An increased intake of vegetables has also been shown to promote cardiovascular health and prevent cellular damage. A study conducted at Harvard University in Boston, Massachusetts, reported that a diet high in vegetables, fruits, nuts, and whole grains improved blood flow and prevented damage to the cells that line the arteries in a group of men with high cholesterol. In this study, increased fruit and vegetable consumption was also found to protect individuals with type 2 diabetes against heart attack, a potential complication of the disease. As for high cholesterol, there's no better way to fight it than with vegetables and fruit. Both are high in fiber, which is known to effectively lower undesirable LDL serum cholesterol levels.

Vitamin C, which is abundant in fresh fruits and vegetables, is an antioxidant that has long been credited with the ability to help protect against cold and infectious diseases. A study reported in the March 3, 2001, issue of *The Lancet* shows that higher blood levels of vitamin C, resulting from a diet high in fruits and vegetables, are also associated with a reduced risk of death from all causes, including heart disease and stroke. Although this study focused on subjects' blood levels of vitamin C, its lead author, Dr. Kay-Tee Khaw from University of Cambridge School of Clinical Medicine in Cambridge, U.K., suggested that the other components of a high fruit and vegetable intake, not just vitamin C itself, may also be responsible for the lower mortality.

Lung function also appears to improve with increased fruit and vegetable consumption, especially a higher intake of apples and tomatoes, according to research done at the University of Nottingham, U.K. Both apples and tomatoes have high levels of antioxidants, which protect against free radical damage. A study conducted by researchers from Finland's National Public Health Institute in Helsinki also concluded that flavonoids from apples, notably the flavonoid *quercetin*, played a critical role in decreasing the risk of lung cancer.

Despite these strong indicators that eating more fruits and vegetables is associated with overall better health, reduced degenerative disease, and lower mortality rates, few Americans have actually increased their intake during the past several years, according to the American Heart Association's 2002 Heart and Stroke Statistical Update. So, as a society, we still have lots of work to do in improving our diet and, by extension, our health. Perhaps we have yet to learn new ways of enjoying our fruits and veggies.

Giving Your Health a Juice Boost

One of the best ways in which to add fruits and vegetables to the diet is with fresh juices. This is, in fact, an effective nutritional shortcut. Just consider the powerful nutrition in two pounds of fresh, raw carrots: 80,000 IU of vitamin A in the form of beta carotene and other carotenoids, along with significant amounts of vitamin C, calcium, magnesium, potassium, and phosphorus. Of course, we wouldn't eat two pounds of raw carrots at any one meal, or even in a single day. But if we were to extract the juice from this amount of carrots (about three cups), we could easily drink, digest, and assimilate it.

That's the major benefit of juicing—we can take in high concentrations of nutrients from raw vegetables and fruits without burdening the digestive system. Drinking fresh juices is recommended in several Cayce readings. Perhaps the most remarkable effect reported by those who have added juices to their diet is an increase in physical energy and mental clarity. Normally, the digestive process takes up more than half the body's available energy. However, since the nutrients in juice are so quickly absorbed, this energy is freed up while the body is richly nourished.

Fresh fruit and vegetable juices supply an abundance of vitamins, minerals, bioflavonoids, and other phytochemicals that help to protect cellular integrity. The enzymes present in fresh juices enhance the assimilation of these nutrients. Cooking and heating foods to about 118°F destroys enzymes, but juicing leaves them intact. Freshly prepared juice is nutritionally superior to bottled juice, which is almost always pasteurized—a process that inhibits enzyme activity to extend shelf life.

Almost any vegetable or fruit is suitable for juicing. Carrot and apple juice are all-time favorites that can be enjoyed on their own or as a base to mix with other juices, such as greens, beetroot, or ginger. Potassium-rich celery is another popular flavor that combines well with stronger tastes. Dark–green leafy vegetables such as kale, watercress, and parsley are an excellent source of chlorophyll, vitamins, and minerals, including calcium and magnesium. However, their strong flavor can be overwhelming to the taste buds. Combining them with a milder–tasting juice makes them more palatable.

Several health experts have advised against combining fruit and vegetables juices, but Michael T. Murray, a naturopathic physician and author of *The Complete Book of Juicing*, says there's no scientific basis for this argument. He suggests, however, that anyone who experiences discomfort from such combinations should avoid them. In general, fruits tend to have a cleansing effect, while vegetables supply nutrients that help build the body.

Some juices also have medicinal value. A favorite is cranberry. Several studies have shown cranberries and cranberry juice to be effective in the prevention and treatment of urinary tract infections, but the jury is still out on the specific substance or mechanism responsible for the popular berry's medicinal effect. Certain chemical compounds in cranberries appear to prevent bacteria, especially E. coli, from adhering to the lining of the bladder and urethra. Some researchers believe that this is due to an increased acidity of the urine following cranberry consumption, while others suggest that the cranberry's acids are not sufficiently concentrated in urine to be solely responsible for this beneficial effect. Most likely it is the special synergistic effect of several substances that makes the cranberry such an effective remedy for urinary tract infections.

Recent research conducted at the University of Scranton in Scranton, Pennsylvania, showed that cranberries contain unusually high concentrations of phenols, which are disease–fighting antioxidants. Phenols are also found in other fruits, but out of nineteen commonly consumed fruits, the cranberry had the highest phenol content. Cranberries are also rich in vitamin C, which helps the body to fight off infections.

Clearly, cranberries are one of Mother Nature's superfoods—a special concentration of powerful nutrients and phytochemicals so well combined that scientists still have not been totally successful in decoding its medicinal secrets.

Because cranberries and their juice have an extremely sour taste, traditional cranberry recipes often call for sweeteners, and commercial cranberry drinks are diluted with other fruit juices. If you're using cranberry juice for medicinal purposes, however, it's best to drink it pure, diluted only with water. Ideally, juice the fresh cranberries at home, dilute with 50 percent pure water, and drink immediately. Alternatively, look for 100 percent pure cranberry juice in natural food stores. If you find even the water dilution unpalatable, try adding pure apple juice or grape juice.

To make fresh juices at home, you'll need a juicer. A high-quality juicer is an investment in your good health. Don't confuse juicers with blenders or food processors, which simply purée the food without separating the juice from the fiber. Juicers extract the juice from fiber of a vegetable or fruit, "unlocking" the nutrients and making them available for easy assimilation. Blenders can, however, be used for mixing bananas, which are too soft to juice, with fresh juices from other fruit to create smoothies in a wide variety of flavors.

For maximum benefit, it's best to consume a wide variety of juices from different types of fruits and vegetables. Just as one vegetable or fruit can't supply all the nourishment the body needs from plants, so one type of juice only provides a partial spectrum of nutrients. Organic fruits and vegetables grown in nutrient-rich soil yield a more nourishing juice and better flavor.

Ideally, fresh juices should be enjoyed as part of a healthy diet, and not merely as a substitute. Eating whole fruits and vegetables is still important because they supply valuable fiber. For best results, drink the juice before meals to optimize absorption.

When Less Is Better

A step that would also benefit many people is to simply eat less. According to a 2001 study by the United States Department of Agriculture (USDA), many Americans are eating multiple serving-sizes of foods such as French fries and pasta at their meals, and this may be contributing to the sharp increase in obesity rates. In several Cayce readings, it is suggested that some people may need to eat less. A middle-aged man who repeatedly consulted Cayce about matters relating to health and diet and who asked, once again, in reading 294–173: *"What change in diet would be best for [the] body now?"* was given this simple advice: *"Don't eat too much!"* In a previous reading, this man had been told that the conditions of congestion in his digestive and assimilating system were caused by excessive eating.

Eating less may indeed help us to live longer, according to a study conducted at the National Institute on Aging (NIA) in Baltimore, Maryland. Dr. Mark A. Lane's research showed that a reduced–calorie diet may prevent several chronic diseases, including cancer, heart disease, and endometriosis. Several previous studies have also shown that cutting calories can increase longevity. In the NIA study, restricting calories appeared to have the strongest impact on diseases that involve abnormal cell growth, such as cancer and endometriosis. Other research has shown that cutting calories protects brain cells from the decline that comes with aging, including from degenerative diseases such as Alzheimer's and Parkinson's disease.

Perhaps reducing our caloric intake could be as simple as cutting out some of our nutrient–low sugary snacks. Studies have revealed that snacking rates in U.S. youth have risen steadily over a twenty–year period from 1980 to 2000. Because sugary snacks contribute mostly "empty" calories, they leave the body hungry for nourishment, causing us to eat more "on the rebound." In addition, refined sugar depletes minerals and vitamins, ultimately increasing requirements for these essential nutrients.

Many snacks, including pretzels, potato chips, corn chips, and cookies, are starchy foods. Starches are complex carbohydrates such as bread, pasta, dried beans and peas, corn, rice, and potatoes. Whenever starches are refined, as in white bread and pasta, their nutrient value is considerably reduced. The Cayce readings suggest that no more than one starchy food should be eaten at the same meal. This means, for instance, that potatoes, pasta, or bread should not be combined with rice, and vice versa. The readings say that an excess of starches has a detrimental effect on the glandular system, which means that the entire metabolism would suffer from too many starchy foods in the diet. Modern research tends to confirm this fact. For instance, the excessive con-

sumption of starchy foods has been associated with a greater incidence
of cancer, especially breast cancer. In 2002, researchers from the Dana-
Farber Cancer Institute, Brigham and Women's Hospital and the Harvard
School of Public Health in Boston also found that a diet high in refined
starches increased women's risk of developing pancreatic cancer.

When grains are incorporated into the diet, they should always be
whole and unrefined. The Cayce readings recommend whole wheat
bread or a well-cooked cereal, such as a gruel made of steel-cut oats, as
wholesome breakfast foods. Whole grains are high in fiber. They also
supply important vitamins and minerals.

Numerous studies have linked whole grain consumption to a lower
risk of heart disease. Research published in the September 27, 2000, issue of *The Journal of the American Medical Association* also showed that eating whole grains lowers the risk of stroke. In other medical studies, patients
who ate whole grains had lower blood sugar levels and decreased insulin concentrations. And a study conducted by researchers of the University of Minnesota in Minneapolis concluded that those who ate
whole grains had a lower risk of death from heart disease and cancer.

A reading that Edgar Cayce gave in 1943 for a thirty-year-old woman
provides a concise summary of a basic whole foods diet: *"In the diets keep
closer to those foods that are easily assimilated; whole grains, plenty of fruits and
vegetables, not too much of meats but plenty of sea foods and fowl—these are preferable for the body."* (2957-1)

Beware of Mainstream "Health Foods"

Today's supermarket shelves are brimming with items catering to the
popular misconception that a healthy diet is largely determined by reduced values of calories, cholesterol, and saturated fats. Catch phrases
such as "cholesterol-free" and "no saturated fats" have dazzled unsus-
pecting consumers eager to keep their arteries clear and their bodies
slim and fit.

An inspection of labels, however, reveals that the substituted ingredients are often more harmful than their supposedly unhealthy counterparts. Let's take a closer look at some of the "health foods" typically
found in supermarkets:

- **"Low–Fat" Breakfast Cereal.** One brand proudly claims to contain "73 percent less fat than oatmeal." If we hadn't previously thought of oatmeal as fattening, we now will! Yet, the product contains added vegetable oil. Vegetable oil is unsaturated and therefore good for you, right? Right, but only if the oil is unrefined and mechanically extracted under the exclusion of light, air, and heat. It must then be refrigerated and consumed within weeks of pressing.

All other commercial vegetable oils, including the popular canola oil, are highly processed and treated with toxic chemicals during extraction and refining. These oils are chemically unstable and vulnerable to rancidity. Quick to deteriorate, these oils produce harmful free radicals, associated with degenerative disease and premature aging.

Oatmeal, with its high fiber content and natural fats, supports metabolic function and overall health. Clearly, it would be the healthier choice! Edgar Cayce recommended steel–cut oats, thoroughly cooked, as an excellent food for the morning meal.

- **"Heart–Healthy" Margarine.** For decades, consumers have been misguided by claims that margarine, made from vegetable oils, is a healthier alternative to butter with its saturated fat content. But how do liquid vegetable oils assume the texture of margarine? It's done through hydrogenation, a process which hardens oils artificially, causing further molecular damage. Hydrogenated oils contain trans–fatty acids (TFAs)—chemically altered molecules that disrupt enzyme function and other metabolic processes in the body. Clinical studies have shown that TFAs raise serum cholesterol levels and contribute to cardiovascular disease.

In response to increasing consumer concerns about TFAs, some margarine producers have eliminated hydrogenated oils from their product. Instead, they've added saturated oils such as palm oil or palm kernel oil to harden the margarine and make it spreadable. Unrefined palm oil and palm kernel oil are actually good for you, but their refined counterparts in margarine are not. The fact remains that margarine is an unhealthy processed fat made from rancid, chemically treated oils. Butter from pasture–fed cows, or olive oil, often recommended by Cayce, are much better choices. Extra virgin olive oil is best, because it is guaranteed to be cold-pressed and unrefined.

• **"Cholesterol–Free" Crackers and Granola Bars.** These, along with most commercial breads, cakes, cookies, and pastries, frequently contain vegetable shortening—a processed fat blended with hydrogenated oils. In addition, such products are often high in sugar, which is an "empty-calorie" food. Sugar disrupts the immune system, metabolism, and glandular balance, and promotes yeast overgrowth. Like refined and processed fats, sugar contributes to cellular damage and heart disease.

High serum levels of undesirable LDL cholesterol may indicate that cellular damage already exists, since cholesterol lines the arteries to provide antioxidant protection against free radical damage caused by processed foods. Excess cholesterol has also been associated with low thyroid function, which in turn is aggravated by high sugar consumption. In other words, sugar promotes the very condition that consumers are hoping to prevent by purchasing "cholesterol-free" snacks!

High-fiber diets rich in fruits, vegetables, and whole grains, on the other hand, have been shown in several studies to lower LDL cholesterol levels. Research conducted at the University of Western Ontario in London, Canada, also showed that drinking three glasses of orange juice a day increases the "good" HDL cholesterol and lowers the ratio between HDL and the "bad" LDL cholesterol. Edgar Cayce often recommended citrus fruits or their juices as breakfast foods, emphasizing, however, that citrus fruits should never be taken at the same time as cereals, except whole wheat toast in small amounts.

Other foods that have been shown to help reduce LDL cholesterol are the macadamia nut, high in monounsaturated fat, and antioxidant-rich cocoa, the compound that gives chocolate its deep, rich flavor.

• **"Low–Calorie" Salad Dressings.** Most low-calorie dressings contain unhealthy substances such as refined vegetable oils, sugar, monosodium glutamate (MSG), and propylene glycol. MSG can trigger sensitivities and migraine headaches in susceptible individuals. Propylene glycol is used industrially to protect machinery from freezing over in winter. It's also found in brake fluid and other mechanical oils. As a food additive, it keeps salad dressings emulsified without the calories of natural oils.

Would consumers still be as eager to save a few calories if they realized that they are dressing their salad greens with antifreeze? Far better if they'd taken a few minutes to make their own dressing with olive oil or a natural mayonnaise. Extra virgin olive oil has long been considered a health food, and new medical studies are proving this claim to be true. The consumption of olive oil has been shown to reduce the risk of developing arthritis, colon cancer, and high blood pressure. A study published in the March 27, 2000, issue of the *Archives of Internal Medicine* showed that some patients who were taking medication for high blood pressure were able to reduce and even eliminate the medication after replacing other fats in their diet with more olive oil. The authors of this study suggested that this may be due to the fact that olive oil contains polyphenols, which are antioxidant compounds that may aid in dilating arteries and thereby in reducing blood pressure.

With salad dressings, as with other foods, it's always best to stick to the natural, unrefined product. Most important, read the label, even in health food stores. And remember that the healthiest foods don't come in a package—they grow on land, on trees, and in the sea!

The Value of Ancestral Diets: A Question of Whole Foods, Digestion, and Assimilation

Some nutritionists argue that our bodies are genetically programmed to thrive on foods which were prevalent in the diet of our ancestors. Research has shown that traditional diets around the world protect ethnic folk from the major killer diseases—cancer and arteriosclerosis—which have become rampant in the industrialized world. The question then is, should we track down our genetic lineage and adopt the diet of our great-grandparents? Would this help to prevent allergies and food intolerances because we would only be eating foods that we can readily digest and assimilate?

While the idea holds appeal, many people would find themselves in conflict if their paternal and maternal ancestors had different ethnic origins. If your grandmother was from southern Italy and your grandfather from northern China, what foods should you put on the dinner table, especially if your spouse brings yet another set of genes to the mix?

A close-up look at ancestral diets reveals that their health benefits are largely found in their commonalities:

- natural whole foods which are locally and seasonally available, as recommended in the Cayce readings;
- foods that are high in enzymes, either because they are fresh and raw, or because they have been naturally preserved through fermentation;
- natural, unrefined fats such as butter, olive oil, and coconut oil.

The traditional Eskimo diet makes for an interesting case study. Even though the Inuit traditionally lived mostly on fatty animal foods, including different species of marine animals, fish, and fish roe and few, if any, vegetables or fruit, they had virtually no heart disease? Why? Given the lack of local plant foods, it might be surprising that the traditional Eskimo diet consisted largely of raw foods. Much of the Inuit's meats, including organ meats, were eaten fresh and raw or frozen, but not cooked. As unappetizing as eating raw meat may seem to the western palate, it was the Eskimo's way of ensuring that he ingested an adequate supply of enzymes to help him digest his food. He even stored his meat in such a way that it would undergo *autolysis*, a process that partially predigests the meat and preserves it at the same time. Predigested foods are high in enzymes and are readily assimilated.

So what to do if your ancestral heritage is Inuit and you now live in California, Virginia, or Texas? Should you eat raw meat and forego vegetables and fruit? Hardly. The consumption of store-bought raw meat is simply not safe, and autolyzed meat not readily available. You need also consider that you live in a different climate and environment. You are less likely to be physically active than your ancestors, even if you exercise regularly. This means that you should eat fewer acid-forming foods, such as meat, and more alkaline-forming foods, such as fruits and vegetables, which also supply plenty of enzymes when eaten raw. In addition, you can incorporate into your diet those foods which offer benefits similar to those found in the traditional Inuit diet.

Lactic-acid fermented foods, for instance, are partially predigested through enzyme action. Yogurt, kefir, and buttermilk are lactic-acid fermented dairy foods which have traditionally been consumed by ethnic groups known for their extraordinary sturdiness and longevity. Although mandatory pasteurization and homogenization have robbed us of the benefits of enzyme-rich raw milk and dairy products, we can still enjoy cultured milk products, in which enzyme action is restored. People of different ethnic backgrounds who are unable to digest regular milk find that fermented milks give them no such problems.

The regular consumption of lactic-acid fermented milk products such as yogurt helps to recolonize the intestinal mucosa with beneficial bacteria, important for the assimilation of nutrients. The Cayce readings recommended yogurt *". . . as an active cleanser through the colon and intestinal system. This would be most beneficial, not only purifying the alimentary canal but adding the vital forces necessary to enable those portions of the system to function in the nearer normal manner."* (1542-1)

Yogurt is especially helpful after treatment with prescription drugs, notably antibiotics, which deplete the beneficial bacteria in the intestinal tact. Modern researchers have shown that yogurt benefits the immune system and may reduce the rate of antibiotic-associated diarrhea. Study results published in the September 1, 2000, issue of *Science* also showed that the beneficial bacteria in the intestinal tract lining may block the body's immune system from causing inflammation in the gut.

The health benefits of natural fermentation are also known in traditional Asian cuisine, where cultured soy products such as miso, tempeh, and natto are popular. Many vegetables can be lactic-acid fermented, including cabbage (the *sauerkraut* of northern and eastern Europe), carrots, radishes, and beets. Traditionally, they are prepared by shredding and mashing the veggies to squeeze out the juice, mixing the pulp and juice with salt and water, then packing everything tightly in a Mason jar and allowing it to stand at room temperature for several days. The naturally present lactic-acid bacteria then initiate the fermentation process, converting the sugars and starches into lactic acid, which helps to restore a healthy bowel flora and destroys putrefactive bacteria in the intestines. Commercially prepared lactic-acid fermented vegetables are available in many natural food stores. Be sure to buy an unpasteurized product.

Unless specific intolerances are present, these foods are nourishing and health-giving for people of all ethnic backgrounds.

Many traditional diets also rely on soaking, sprouting, and sour-leavening to make foods more nutritious and easier to digest. These practices help to break down the phytates in grains and seeds, which otherwise interfere with the absorption of minerals. Sprouting also multiplies the vitamin content of plant foods.

What traditional diets lack is refined flour and sugar, overcooked foods devoid of enzymes, pasteurized milk and cheese, and processed, hydrogenated vegetable oils. When our digestive system revolts and we find that we cannot tolerate certain grains or dairy, it is not necessarily because these foods were absent from our great-grandparents' diet. Rather, it is the modern, processed versions of these foods that are indigestible and cause illness. A return to a natural whole foods diet is the answer, whatever our ancestral lineage.

Who Needs Nutritional Supplements?

Forty percent of Americans take a nutritional supplement at least occasionally, spending up to $1.7 billion each year on vitamins and minerals. Is this money well spent, or is it literally going down the drain?

Most nutritionists would agree with the Cayce readings which say that the nutrients the body needs should ideally come from fresh, natural, whole foods. Cayce was adamant in the recommendation that " . . . *nature is much better yet than science!*" (759-13) Yet, several individuals who received readings from Cayce were told to take specific vitamin and mineral preparations. In cases where the diet is less than optimal, food intake is restricted or simply does not meet an individual's biochemical requirements, a nutritional supplement, taken orally or with medical help by injection into the bloodstream, can indeed make the difference between health and illness.

Consider the study done with a group of patients in western New York who suffered from severe myopathy, a muscle disorder which had weakened them to such an extent that they were confined to wheelchairs. A team of doctors from State University of New York at Buffalo and Kaleida Health in Buffalo put them on a high–potency vitamin D supplement. Within six weeks, all study participants reported notice-able improvement, including a resolution of pain and a restoration of normal muscle strength.

Four patients became fully mobile, and the fifth also became mobile. In each case, weakness and immobility had previously been attributed to other causes, including old age, diabetic neuropathy, or general de-bility. But it was a simple nutrient—vitamin D—which gave these people the strength to get out of their wheelchairs and walk!

Vitamin D, a fat–soluble vitamin which helps the body assimilate calcium and other nutrients required for healthy bones, muscles, and nerves, is produced in the body through the interaction of the ultravio-let rays of the sun with certain chemicals in the fatty tissue under the skin. Food sources of vitamin D are fish and fish liver oils, and eggs and dairy products.

Vitamin D deficiency is widespread in North America and other geo-graphical areas where people don't get enough sunshine on a regular basis. Poor nutrition, fat–restricted diets, and intestinal malabsorption are other contributing factors. When Edgar Cayce was asked what changes in civilization were the causes for vitamin D deficiency, he an-swered: *"The tendency to have less sunshine activity, or less activity in the sunshine, and the taking of more foods that are not close to nature."* (658–11) More than half a century later, Cayce's words are echoed in several medical studies, including one reported in the December 2001 issue of the *European Jour-nal of Clinical Nutrition*, in which researchers found that during the winter, many women in Canada had insufficient blood levels of vitamin D de-spite drinking vitamin–D fortified milk or taking a dietary supplement of vitamin D. The group of patients in western New York needed more vitamin D than was normally supplied by diet. Who would expect that taking a single vitamin could make someone get out of a wheelchair and walk?

In another medical study, researchers found that a vitamin–like sub-stance, coenzyme Q10 (CoQ10), could successfully treat some cases of hereditary ataxia, a disease characterized by an inability to coordinate voluntary muscle movements. Some ataxia patients have problems with balance or speech, while others suffer from seizures. CoQ10 aids oxygen utilization in the body. In this study, a team of researchers at Columbia University's College of Physicians and Surgeons in New York identified six patients with hereditary ataxia whose CoQ10 levels were significantly below normal. Five of the six could not walk. After taking a high-potency CoQ10 supplement, all patients showed dramatic improvement in strength and well-being and were able to walk, although they required assistance, for instance a rolling walker.

Although it may seem surprising that a single nutrient such as a vitamin should have so much healing power, it is consistent with Edgar Cayce's definition of vitamins as the *"creative forces working with the body-energies for the renewing of the body!"* (3511-1) This underscores the importance of nutrition, and of vitamins, in restoring good health.

If nutritional supplements can bring about such a dramatic improvement in the condition of those who are seriously disabled by their nutritional deficiencies, can we imagine how many minor aches and pains we would be able to take care of with nutrition and supplements in those of us who simply feel unwell, fatigued, or unhappy as a result of less than optimal intake of certain nutrients?

The question is, how can we determine which nutrient is in short supply, and whether it can be supplied by diet alone, or whether a supplement is necessary? A good rule of thumb is to try a natural whole foods diet first and note if your specific condition or general health improves. If no improvement is seen within a couple of months, add a whole-foods concentrate or a good-quality multiple vitamin and mineral supplement. If this is not effective, it may be worth your while to consult a qualified nutritionist or naturopathic physician to help you identify the specific supplements that would most likely replenish your body's store of the nutrients that are inadequately present. You may be surprised at the difference that appropriate supplementation can make in your overall health and well-being!

The Cayce readings generally suggested that nutritional supplements should not be taken on a permanent basis so that the body would not lose the ability to synthesize nutrients from foods. The summer months, when you spend more time outdoors, or when you go on vacation, might be a good time to take a break from supplements.

Weight Loss and the Calorie-Counting Myth

The load on Mother Earth is getting heavier. Not only are there more of us to carry, we weigh more, too. Worldwide, the number of over-weight people is estimated at 1.2 billion. More than 39 percent of adults in the U.S. are overweight and an additional 20 percent are considered obese—excessively fat. Obesity is more than a cosmetic problem. Obese people are at higher risk for degenerative conditions such as high blood pressure, diabetes, heart disease, arthritis, and cancer. Obesity statistics hold interesting clues. While large population groups in Third World countries are malnourished due to lack of food, an equally large num-ber of people in developed nations are malnourished because of exces-sive food consumption.

Is that not a contradiction in terms? Choice of foods is the key. It is also the reason why the estimated 30 percent of North American adults who are on a weight–loss program at any given time are often unsuc-cessful in keeping excess pounds off beyond the duration of their par-ticular diet.

If we restrict food intake for a time and then resume our old habits of eating processed and refined foods devoid of nutrients, we effectively starve an already malnourished body. Counting calories might further our math skills, but will get us nowhere nutritionally. What we need to look at are the types of foods that are eaten and how they are digested, assimilated, and metabolized. If any components of good nutrition are compromised, metabolic function will be impaired and weight and tox-ins will accumulate.

Detoxification must be the first step in any weight–loss program. Our strongest ally in the effort to detoxify is water. Drink at least eight to ten glasses of filtered, distilled, or spring water each day. Water can also help to curb appetite. In fact, a hungry feeling may be the body's first call for water, often misinterpreted for food hunger. Whenever hungry, try drinking a large glass of water first. You may find that you no longer desire food. Even if the hunger returns, you'll be inclined to eat less at the meal that follows. Adding a few drops of fresh lemon juice boosts water's cleansing potential.

Fruits and fruit juices are also helpful. Grapes, in particular, are ideal for any weight–loss program. They have a cleansing effect on the system, promoting good digestion and assimilation, as well as glandular coordination. Grape juice, diluted 2:1 with water, to be taken before meals and at bedtime, was repeatedly recommended by Cayce for individuals suffering from obesity. Pineapple juice is high in the enzyme bromelain, which aids digestion and has been shown to promote weight loss.

Achieving and maintaining one's ideal body weight is essentially a function of metabolism—of how foods are burned and utilized in the body. Once toxins are eliminated and digestion is improved, we can keep our metabolism well–tuned with a natural whole foods diet and a healthy lifestyle. Here are some important suggestions:

• Avoid excessively starchy foods, especially processed carbohydrates and white–flour products. These are the "empty calories" that cause weight gain in the first place. Build your meals around vegetables and fruits, which supply vitamins, minerals, fiber, enzymes, and a host of phytochemicals and nutraceuticals that aid in balancing the metabolism.

• Eat more raw foods, which not only provide superior nutrition, but also the enzymes necessary for their own digestion. The cooking process destroys these naturally occurring enzymes, forcing the pancreas to produce more internal digestive enzymes. Aim to have at least one completely raw meal each day, or eat a raw salad with a cooked meal twice a day.

• Eat two or three servings of high–quality protein each day. Protein is required for proper metabolic function and endocrine balance. Free–range eggs, fowl, fish, and dairy products (ideally fermented, such as yogurt or kefir) provide excellent protein. Vegetarian sources are combinations of legumes, grains, seeds, and nuts.

• Add some green tea to your diet. A study at the University of Geneva in Switzerland showed that certain compounds in organic green tea may promote weight loss by increasing thermogenesis (the burning of body fat).

• Nourish your thyroid—a master gland in the endocrine system which determines a number of biochemical reactions, including protein synthesis and the rate at which the body burns fat. To function optimally, the thyroid needs a continuous supply of iodine, an essential mineral and a vital constituent of the hormones produced by the thyroid. Seafoods and sea vegetables such as kelp, dulse, kombu, nori, and arame are particularly rich in iodine and should form a regular part of the diet. Kelp and dulse are also available in tablet form in health food stores. Asparagus, watercress, Swiss chard, parsley, and turnip greens also contain iodine. Other nutrients important for thyroid function include zinc, copper, selenium, and the B vitamins, notably B6.

• Know your fat facts. The popular assumption that all fats are bad and that any fat eaten will automatically transform into body fat is a myth based on misinformation. Some dietary fat is necessary for optimal metabolic function! The type of fat is important, however. Avoid processed, refined vegetable oils (this includes most supermarket brands), hydrogenated fats like margarine, and vegetable shortenings. Use unrefined, cold-pressed vegetable oils like flax seed, walnut, and sunflower instead, but never cook or bake with them, as heat causes them to break down and become toxic. For cooking and baking, use only fats which remain stable at high temperatures, such as butter, extra-virgin olive oil, macadamia nut oil, coconut oil, or palm oil.

Supplementing the diet with flax seed and evening primrose oil provides important essential fatty acids, which encourage weight loss by supporting endocrine function.

Although it is possible to lose weight without exercise, a trim, firm body can only be achieved through physical activity. So go out and walk, run, swim, clean out the garage, or push the vacuum. Anything that gets the body moving will speed up the metabolism and help you to stay slim and healthy!

Salt or No Salt?

Salt has become almost a dirty word in the world of nutrition. Yet, salt is an important nutrient which has been greatly misunderstood. Sodium, the primary constituent of salt, is considered a vital electrolyte mineral, helping to convey energy and the spark of life itself—the electrical charge that is essential for all cellular functions and facilitates muscle contraction and the transmission of nerve impulses.

The chloride in salt promotes the production of hydrochloric acid (HCl) in the stomach. HCl is required for the digestion of proteins and minerals. Many people don't secrete enough HCl, often because of a reaction to stress which creates tension in the solar plexus area, inhibiting HCl. When salt is added to the diet, digestion improves and with it the assimilation of nutrients from other foods. In many traditional diets, salty soups or broths are taken at the beginning of a meal to stimulate digestion.

How strange it is then that in recent times salt has acquired such a poor reputation, being implicated in high blood pressure and several other health problems. When we look at the medical studies that support these claims, however, we find that they have all been carried out with common table salt, made from refined rock salt that has been stripped of its natural mineral balance, reducing it to 99 percent sodium chloride. The rest is additives—bleaching and free–flowing agents, stabilizers, and aluminum compounds.

Some people believe that simply using sea salt is healthier. However, the same guidelines apply to sea salt as to any other food: when it's refined, it's not a health food. Sea salt that is white, dry, and free–flowing has been highly refined, removing essential minerals and trace elements. Like common table salt, refined sea salt is mostly sodium chloride and contains no other nutrients.

Whole, unrefined sea salt is light–gray in color. Because it is hand–harvested and naturally dried by the sun and air rather than through the artificial heat of a kiln, it retains a moist, lumpy texture. Unprocessed sea salt contains more than eighty essential minerals and trace elements in a complex balance that closely resembles the constituents of human body fluids—blood, lymph, sweat, and tears are all salty.

The essential trace mineral iodine is present in unrefined sea salt in a form that is easily assimilated. Iodine is a vital constituent of the hormones produced by the thyroid gland, which controls several biochemical reactions, including oxygen utilization, protein synthesis, and the rate at which the body burns food. The refining process destroys the iodine in white sea salt. An inorganic form of iodine, most often potassium iodide, is added to refined table salt. However, this type of iodine is not readily assimilated by the body. It passes in the urine quickly, usually within twenty minutes, whereas natural iodine from unrefined sea salt is retained for forty-eight hours—long enough to be utilized by the thyroid. Unlike table salt, unrefined sea salt also supplies the thyroid with other important minerals and trace elements.

The Cayce readings generally advise against the use of common table salt. Instead, the readings recommend kelp salt, deep sea salt, or "health salt" prepared from dried vegetables. Reading 2084–16 says: *"Do use only the health salt or kelp salt or deep sea salt. All of these are of the same characters. But they are better than just that which has been purified, for the general health of many . . ."* Kelp salt is made from the dried and powdered sea vegetable kelp, which is an excellent source of iodine and other minerals. It tends to have a slightly bitter taste, and some find it unpalatable. Unrefined sea salt has a richer flavor than common table salt, thus less is needed to achieve the same full taste and aroma.

If you're still concerned about mainstream nutritionists' call to reduce salt intake to prevent or cure high blood pressure, consider the study by Duke University Medical Center in which a diet high in fresh fruits and vegetables reduced blood pressure in patients with near-normal salt intake to levels previously attainable only with medication. Like unrefined sea salt, vegetables and fruits provide plenty of minerals to balance out the sodium. Just adding a few servings to the daily diet achieves better results than giving up on salt. Unrefined sea salt can even help to normalize blood pressure by breaking down fats and cholesterol in the arteries and promoting good circulation.

Salt-free diets probably cause more health problems than they are touted to correct. Moderate amounts of salt are vital for good health. But the salt that is used must be whole, unrefined, and made by nature itself.

Diet and Cancer

According to researchers who presented their findings at the European Conference on Nutrition and Cancer in Lyon, France, in June 2001, almost one in three cancers could be prevented through a healthier diet.

Cancer develops when cells in the body function abnormally and multiply uncontrollably—a process which eventually leads to tumor growth. A healthy body routinely detects and eliminates abnormal cells. When the immune system is compromised and certain raw materials required for cellular health are not supplied, cancer results.

Research studies consistently demonstrate that individuals with a high intake of certain foods and nutritional supplements are less likely than others to develop specific types of cancer. By ensuring that these nutrients are adequately supplied and assimilated, we can prevent deficiencies that might predispose us to a host of degenerative conditions—including cancer.

It is important to remember that cancer is not a calorie deficiency. In fact, the reverse appears to be the case. Research has shown that countries with the greatest per capita caloric intake have the highest incidence and mortality rates from cancer. Citizens of these countries often also eat large amounts of refined and processed foods.

White flour, refined sugar, refined grains, and refined vegetable oils are nutrient robbers because the body uses up important enzymes, vitamins, and minerals to break down and eliminate them. It is thus possible to eat large amounts of food and even put on weight while the body starves for vital nutrients.

Let's look at some of the nutritional deficiencies that are often involved in the development of cancer:

Enzyme chemistry.   Enzymes are organic catalysts necessary for every biochemical reaction in the body, including the process of digestion. When raw foods are eaten, the enzymes they naturally contain facilitate digestion, reducing the demand on the body's pancreatic secretions. Cooked foods are devoid of enzymes, as they are destroyed by heat. The long-term consumption of cooked foods creates a chronic enzyme deficiency, which predisposes the body to cancerous conditions.

Dr. Edward Howell, author of *Enzyme Nutrition*, says that "there is abundant laboratory proof of profoundly disturbed enzyme chemistry in cancer." Enzyme-rich foods and enzyme supplements are important factors in both the prevention and treatment of cancer.

Lactic-acid fermented foods—such as natural sauerkraut, yogurt, kefir, and buttermilk—also supply valuable enzymes. As was discussed earlier, they stimulate the production of beneficial bacteria in the intestinal tract, thus promoting the proper digestion and assimilation of foods and the elimination of disease–causing organisms and carcinogens.

Miso—a naturally fermented food made from soybeans—is valued as a medicinal food in the macrobiotic diet, which is widely regarded as an effective dietary regimen for healing cancer and other degenerative conditions.

Antioxidant action. Nutritional deficiencies of the antioxidant vitamins A, B–complex, C, E, and the carotenoids (especially beta–carotene, the precursor form of vitamin A) are often associated with cancer. This is because the body needs these antioxidants to destroy free radicals, which are byproducts of normal metabolism. If free radicals are uncontrolled, they encourage the development of cancerous tumors.

Lycopene, a carotenoid found in tomatoes, has been the subject of several research studies in recent years. A high intake of tomato products is associated with a reduced risk for cancer; especially of the prostate, lung, and stomach.

Other foods rich in antioxidants are various types of berries and raw or unpasteurized honey. The Cayce readings recommend raw, unpasteurized honey, preferably taken with the honeycomb, as a healing food for a variety of ailments, including anemia, arthritis, diabetes, toxemia, and psoriasis.

Protection through minerals. Mineral deficiencies—notably calcium, selenium, zinc, iodine and germanium—are also common in cancer patients. Selenium, in particular, has been shown to have cancer–protective properties. Research conducted at the University of Hawaii in Honolulu in 2002 also showed that a high intake of calcium may lower women's risk of developing ovarian cancer.

A convenient way to increase mineral intake is by adding sea vegetables to the diet on a regular basis. A variety of dried sea veggies can be found in the macrobiotic section of health food stores. Some seaweeds, such as kelp and dulse, are also available in powder, tablet, or liquid extract form.

Deep–green and orange–colored vegetables and fruits are excellent sources of antioxidant nutrients and should be part of the diet every day. The Cayce readings emphasized the importance of including these foods in the diet on a regular basis. Deep–green and orange–colored fruits and veggies have the additional benefit of contributing alkaline–forming elements, thus ensuring that the body's pH balance is kept slightly alkaline for optimal metabolic function. As discussed earlier, a diet that is 80 percent alkaline forming ensures that no acidic residues are allowed to accumulate in the body.

Fabulous fruits and veggies.   Cruciferous vegetables—which include broccoli, cauliflower, cabbage, Brussels sprouts, and kale—have also been associated with lowered cancer risk, especially of the stomach, colon, and breast. This is due to the action of the plants' indoles, which block the proliferation of cancer cells. In 2002, researchers at the Ohio State University also found that regular intake of berries, notably strawberries and black raspberries, had a powerful cancer–inhibiting effect. While this is encouraging news, it's important to remember that berries and other seasonal fruits are best eaten as that—*in season*. Ideally, our food should also be organic. Otherwise, we risk ingesting a food that's been heavily sprayed with pesticides and quite likely also has been modified through genetic engineering, which refers to the merging of genes from plants, animals, viruses, and bacteria in ways that do not occur in nature. For instance, the DNA from an arctic fish, such as a flounder, might be spliced into the DNA of a fruit, such as a strawberry, to make it frost–resistant. Our knowledge of the consequences of the genetic engineering of foods is extremely limited, and many scientists are concerned that it may cause irreparable damage, for instance through accidental cross–pollination and the creation of modified viruses and bacteria that may introduce new diseases unknown to the immune systems of humans, animals, and plants.

Essential fatty acids.   A deficiency of essential fatty acids (EFAs) can also put the body at risk for cancer. High–quality natural fats are important for cellular and metabolic health. The integrity of the skin and nervous system, the endocrine and digestive system all depend on an adequate supply of EFAs in the diet. Not only is the typical North American diet low in EFAs, but it is also often loaded with refined, processed, and hydrogenated vegetable oils which disrupt the metabolism and further interfere with the function of EFAs.

Dr. Johanna Budwig successfully used a combination of flax seed oil and quark cheese in the treatment of cancer. Flax seed oil is high in EFAs, especially the important omega-3 type. Fresh nuts and seeds provide high concentrations of EFAs. The Cayce readings repeatedly state that eating one or more almonds each day is an effective way to protect against the development of cancerous tumors. Other sources of EFAs include dark-green leafy vegetables and several types of unrefined, unprocessed vegetable oils available in opaque glass bottles in the refrigerated section of natural food stores.

Water—our most effective medicine.   It's hard to believe, but the health benefits of the most abundant substance in nature—water— are still not widely recognized. Pure water is required for digestion and the elimination of toxins and waste products. We depend on water to deliver nutrients to the cells and for the circulation of blood, lymph, and interstitial fluids. No wonder the metabolism is disrupted when water intake is inadequate! A study reported in the May 6, 1999, issue of the *New England Journal of Medicine* showed that men who drank at least six glasses of water a day cut their risk of bladder cancer in half compared with men who drank less than one glass.

Some studies have also linked heavy meat consumption with cancer. Research reported in the January 2002 issue of the *American Journal of Clinical Nutrition* demonstrated that people who eat large amounts of meat and dairy products have double the risk of stomach cancer and esophageal cancer when compared with people who eat diets high in vegetables, fruits, and whole grains.

Edgar Cayce often told people to restrict their meat intake and to instead build their diet around vegetables and fruits. An 80 percent alkaline-forming diet allows for a considerably smaller portion of meat and dairy products—the moderate amounts that are considered acceptable and healthful in the Cayce diet. The types of meats that were said to be most beneficial in the readings are fish, fowl, and lamb. As for dairy, the readings recommended yogurt and moderate amounts of soft cheese for the normal diet.

Other studies have linked charbroiled meat with cancer risk. The charring of meats which usually occurs during barbecuing and frying results in the formation of carcinogens. The cooking methods recommended in the Cayce readings were baking, roasting, and broiling, while frying was consistently advised against.

Last but not least—an optimistic note about the cancer–preventing properties of grapes, which were often recommended for culinary and medicinal use in the Cayce readings. Researchers from the School of Pharmacy at De Montfort University, Leicester, U.K., have isolated a substance in grapes which is converted in the body to a known anti–cancer agent that can selectively destroy cancer cells. This study confirms previous research about the cancer–inhibiting properties of *resveratrol*, a phenolic compound that also contributes to the health–promoting reputation enjoyed by red wine.

High-Fiber Diet for Diabetes

Diabetes is a leading cause of death in the United States and many other developed countries. It is a chronic degenerative disease in which the body is unable to utilize sugar in the normal manner. In a healthy person, the hormone insulin, secreted by the pancreas, facilitates the transport of blood sugar (glucose) to the cells for use as energy.

In type I diabetes (insulin–dependent juvenile diabetes), the pancreas either makes insufficient amounts of insulin or has ceased insulin production completely. In the more common type II diabetes (non-insulin dependent adult onset diabetes), insulin is still produced, but the body has developed a resistance to the hormone and is unable to absorb glucose for cellular energy.

The body's inability to adequately nourish its cells with glucose often leads to other debilitating conditions such as coronary heart disease, kidney damage, nerve degeneration, and impaired or lost vision and hearing.

Obesity and physical inactivity are known risk factors in the development of type II diabetes. Those who already have this disease need to reduce excess weight and balance glucose in the blood stream by following a diet of natural whole foods and taking appropriate supplements. Even type I diabetics, who depend on regular insulin injections, often find that their need for injected insulin can be reduced through a nutrition and exercise plan which aims at lowering overall blood sugar levels. A study conducted at the University of Ottawa, Canada, in 2001 showed that people who had type 2 diabetes and who undertook a regular exercise program were able to lower glucose levels and found themselves in better health overall. Exercise helps to sensitize cells in the liver and muscles to insulin.

Above all, diabetics must eliminate refined carbohydrates from the diet. Refined sugar and refined grain products, such as white flour, white rice and pasta, and processed foods which contain them, must be avoided. Why? Because refined carbohydrates flood the blood stream with sugar, placing a heavy burden on the pancreas to respond to severe fluctuations in blood sugar levels.

A natural whole foods diet, consisting of fresh vegetables and fruits, high-quality protein, and whole grains, nuts, and seeds, can help to regulate blood sugar levels. The high fiber supplied by such a diet slows the rate of food passage through the intestinal tract and results in a more gradual release of glucose into the blood stream. According to a research report in the September 2000 issue of the *American Journal of Public Health*, a diet emphasizing whole grain products can lower the risk of developing diabetes. A few months earlier, a study reported in *The New England Journal of Medicine* in May 2000 concluded that a high-fiber diet leads to a significant reduction in glucose levels in type II diabetics. One of the medical editors of this study pointed out that the decrease in high blood sugar was comparable to that achieved with an oral diabetes drug.

Over half a century ago, the Cayce readings made similar recommendations for the nutritional management of diabetes by emphasizing a diet based on fresh vegetables and fruits. In addition, the Jerusalem artichoke was recommended to help control blood sugar levels. A gnarled root vegetable that resembles a knotty potato, the Jerusalem artichoke is not botanically related to the more popular globe artichoke. Many holistic health practitioners today recommend Jerusalem artichokes in the dietary management of diabetes. *Inulin*, a soluble fiber found in Jerusalem artichokes, helps to stabilize glucose levels. The Cayce readings suggest that the regular use of Jerusalem artichokes may reduce and even eliminate the need for insulin medication:

Instead of using so much insulin; this can be gradually diminished

and eventually eliminated entirely if there is used in the diet one
Jerusalem artichoke every other day. This should be cooked only in
Patapar paper, preserving the juices and mixing with the bulk of the
artichoke, seasoning this to suit the taste. The taking of the insulin is
habit forming. The artichoke is not habit forming . . .   4023-1

The Jerusalem artichoke may be cooked like a potato, or it can be used in vegetable soups, stews, and casseroles. It can also be juiced or eaten raw, grated in salads.

In addition, appropriate nutritional supplements can help to control blood sugar levels, as well as prevent or diminish many of the degenerative symptoms associated with diabetes. Of particular importance is brewer's yeast, a good source of the biologically active form of chromium, a component of Glucose Tolerance Factor, which supports the action of insulin in moving glucose from the blood stream into the cells. Other important nutrients include digestive enzymes, the B–complex vitamins, vitamin E, and magnesium.

The Cayce readings also recommend spinal adjustments, colon hydrotherapy, and moderate exercise. A regular exercise program, in particular, supports a sound nutrition plan by improving metabolic function—so important for the absorption and assimilation of nutrients.

Nutritional Support for Arthritis

The term arthritis encompasses more than one hundred rheumatic diseases that, to varying degrees, can cause pain, stiffness, and swelling in the joints. Although arthritis is often regarded as a degenerative disease that accompanies aging, it can affect men, women, and children of all ages. More women than men suffer from this condition. The most common form of arthritis is osteoarthritis, also referred to as degenerative joint disease. In this condition, the cartilage covering the ends of bones has begun to wear away, causing bone surfaces to rub together at the joint. The symptoms of osteoarthritis are usually experienced as pain and stiffness in the joints, aggravated by movement and weight bearing.

A more destructive form of arthritis, rheumatoid arthritis, is characterized by inflammation in the synovial membranes of the joints, as well as by bone atrophy. Rheumatoid arthritis is considered an autoimmune disease, in which a faulty immune response causes the body to attack its own cells.

At the start of the millennium, the United Nations launched *The Bone and Joint Decade*, a ten-year international campaign aimed at improving the lives of those afflicted with bone and joint conditions such as arthritis, osteoporosis, and other spinal and musculoskeletal disorders. Two of the goals set for this project are "to empower patients to participate in their own health care" and "to promote cost-effective prevention and treatment."

One of the most effective ways in which arthritis patients can become active participants in their own health care is through nutrition. From a nutritional point of view, arthritis is a deficiency disease. Nutritional deficiencies or imbalances may be due to poor diet, incomplete digestion and assimilation, faulty elimination of toxins, or lack of circulation in the system.

Gastrointestinal problems play a significant role in the development and proliferation of arthritis. The incidence of arthritis is higher in individuals who have been diagnosed with conditions such as colitis, inflammatory bowel disease, parasites, or other intestinal disorders. Any digestive disturbances must be addressed before arthritis can be treated successfully.

A detoxification program is an important first step in restoring healthy bowel function. Cleansing fasts of fresh vegetable juices or clear broths, or mono-diets of fresh apples or grapes for two or three days, help to rid the body of accumulated toxins. Longer fasts should only be undertaken in consultation with a qualified health care practitioner. It is essential during such times to keep the bowels moving to prevent reabsorption of toxins from the colon into the bloodstream. Intestinal bulking agents such as psyllium hulls or flaxseed are helpful, as are enemas and colonic irrigation. Drinking lots of pure water is essential, as water provides the most important medium for the elimination of toxins.

A predominantly alkaline-forming diet, emphasizing vegetables and fruits, is especially important for the arthritic body, which tends to accumulate high levels of uric acid in the tissues. Dark-green leafy and orange-colored vegetables are also rich sources of antioxidants, bioflavonoids, and other phytochemicals which have been shown to reduce symptoms of arthritis. Results of a Greek study reported in the *American Journal of Clinical Nutrition* demonstrate that the Mediterranean diet, high in olive oil and vegetables, offers protection against arthritis.

A number of nutritional supplements are known to reduce pain and inflammation from arthritis:

Gelatin.   Often recommended by Cayce, gelatin promotes the assimilation of nutrients from foods and supplements. It supports calcium metabolism and helps to build healthy bones and joints. Research at the Rippe Lifestyle Institute has found that daily doses of gelatin appear to help ease the pain and disability associated with osteoarthritis of the knee. Individuals taking gelatin were found to show a significant improvement in strength compared to those who did not take gelatin.

Glucosamine sulfate.   This substance, derived from the shells of crab, lobster, and shrimp, helps the body to repair damaged cartilage. A study at the University of Belgium has confirmed the benefits of glucosamine sulfate. Patients who took 1,500 mg daily for three years reported a significant reduction in pain and movement restriction.

Chondroitin sulfate.   This supplement increases the ability of cartilage to act as a shock absorber in the joints by drawing fluid and nutrients into the cartilage tissue. The effectiveness of chondroitin sulfate in the treatment of osteoarthritis is the focus of a major study funded by the National Institutes of Health.

Green tea.   Research conducted at Case Western Reserve University's School of Medicine showed that the consumption of green tea may prevent and reduce the severity of rheumatoid arthritis. The antioxidant action of polyphenols, special chemicals present in green tea, is believed to be responsible for this effect.

Quercetin.   A bioflavonoid which naturally occurs in certain fruits and vegetables, quercetin has an anti-inflammatory effect in rheumatoid arthritis.

Devil's claw root and **feverfew.**   Both herbs have been shown to reduce inflammation and joint pain in arthritis.

Evening primrose oil.   High in gamma-linolenic acid, evening primrose oil helps to reduce inflammation and to correct a deficiency in certain essential fatty acids. Omega–3 fish oils appear to have a similar effect.

Sea Kelp.   This is a rich source of minerals, particularly iodine, which supports the healthy function of the thyroid and the whole glandular system. Endocrine imbalances appear to play a role in arthritis. For instance, women who have taken hormone–replacement therapy for more than five years are twice as likely to develop arthritis than women who have not. The regular consumption of kelp rejuvenates and balances the entire endocrine system. Edgar Cayce often recommended kelp powder as healthier alternative to regular table salt.

In addition to dietary adjustments, several alternative modalities have shown promising results in the treatment of arthritis. Acupuncture, massage, aromatherapy, exercise, and hydrotherapy are effective in reducing symptoms of inflammation, joint pain, and immobility. Sufficient time outdoors in natural sunlight is also important.

Edgar Cayce's recommendations for the treatment of arthritis include Epsom salt baths, massage with peanut oil, and supplementation with Atomidine to balance the endocrine system. Dr. William A. McGarey's excellent book, *Heal Arthritis: Physically-Mentally-Spiritually*, provides a comprehensive outline of these and other holistic therapies.

As in any illness, emotional and spiritual components play an important role in arthritis.

In 1999, a study reported in the *Journal of the American Medical Association* concluded that arthritis patients who, for several days, wrote down their feelings about a stressful event in their lives, saw their symptoms improve dramatically within four months.

The results of this medical study clearly support the concepts that are at the basis of mind/body medicine. Arthritis is a whole–person disease, and only a holistic approach to treatment can bring about true healing.

Methods of Therapeutic Manipulation: A Hands-on Approach to Better Health

As oft as practical have the prayer and the laying on of hands.

Edgar Cayce reading 2606-1

THE TOUCH OF the human hand is a powerful healing agent when applied with love. This touch can relieve pain, relax tension, reassure, console, and comfort. Research has shown that gently holding another's wrist helps to reduce that person's heartbeat and blood pressure. Many physicians unconsciously make use of the relaxing power of touch by gently resting their hand on the patient's shoulder during an examination or treatment. Touch promotes a baby's growth and development. In a clinical study with prematurely born infants, those who were gently stroked for forty-five minutes a day gained considerably more weight than those who were not stroked, even though both groups were fed the same amount of calories. Touching promotes the release of the brain chemical *beta-endorphin*, an endorphin of the pituitary gland that has considerable analgesic effects and also appears to promote growth and development. In *The Edgar Cayce Handbook for Health Through Drugless*

Therapy, authors Dr. Harold J. Reilly and Ruth Hagy Brod explain the relaxing effect of touch: "In humans, quiet stroking of different parts of the body brings about a relaxing semihypnotic feeling that has a more favorable effect on the nervous system than tranquilizers and sleeping pills—with none of the detrimental after-effects."

Stroking and touching are wonderful tools for healing. Yet, as a society, we seem to be afraid of touching or being touched. We fear that we might offend someone, or that we might transgress boundaries by reaching out in touch to others. Perhaps we're afraid of spreading or "catching" germs. In the healing arts, however, therapies that employ touch have enjoyed increasing popularity in recent years. Methods of therapeutic manipulation are thriving in a world that is tired of an excessively cold and sterile environment, such as a hospital or other medical facility. We long to be touched again, and we hunger for that transfer of energy that takes place when a healing hand reaches out to another with love.

There are many different healing modalities that employ touch in a systematic and therapeutic manner. Of these, chiropractic and massage are most easily recognized today. Others, such as Polarity Therapy, Rolfing, and the Trager method, are gaining increasing public recognition. Therapeutic Touch, a system that is based on the laying on of hands but which, surprisingly, works through subtle manipulation of a person's energy field, has been incorporated into many physiotherapy programs in hospitals and nursing homes. Cayce reading 281-4 states that *"there are those that need the body vibrations each day, that these may be made whole by the laying on of hands . . . "*

In this chapter, we will review some of the most popular methods of therapeutic manipulation.

Chiropractic

Chiropractic is the largest drugless healing profession. The word "chiropractic" is derived from the Greek words "cheir" and "praktkos," meaning "done by hand." A chiropractic physician uses his or her hands to identify and correct misalignments, or "subluxations," of the spinal vertebrae—the twenty-four small bones that surround and protect the spinal cord. The spinal nerves, which are an extension of the spinal cord, pass between the vertebrae and branch out to every part of the body, including the organs, glands, bones, and muscles. When the vertebrae rotate, tilt, or otherwise get out of alignment, pressure is placed on the spinal nerves, restricting their ability to conduct nerve impulses. Therefore, the tissues or organs that are served by the impinged nerves do not receive the nerve energy required for optimal health. This causes the affected tissues and organs to weaken and become susceptible to attack by bacteria and other organisms. If the condition remains uncorrected, such tissues and organs may ultimately degenerate and develop pathological symptoms.

Chiropractic, therefore, treats more than just back pain or joint problems. When subluxations of the vertebrae are corrected and proper nerve flow is restored through chiropractic adjustments of the spinal column, it is not uncommon for seemingly unrelated organic symptoms to disappear as well.

The art and science of chiropractic dates back to 1895, when Daniel David Palmer, a longtime student of physiology and anatomy, established the theory and specific techniques of chiropractic. Palmer had developed this theory after meeting a janitor who became deaf after suffering an injury to his upper spine. When Palmer examined the janitor's spine, he discovered a misaligned vertebrae in the area of the spine where the injury had occurred. Palmer then applied a specific thrust to realign the vertebrae, with the result that the janitor also regained his hearing.

D.D. Palmer based his healing philosophy on the concept that residing in all living beings is an innate intelligence which flows through the central nervous system, delivering energy to the tissues and organs and coordinating vital body functions in the process. If the flow of this innate intelligence is impeded, pathological conditions result. The task of the chiropractor, therefore, is to skillfully apply the appropriate thrusts to the vertebrae that would realign the spinal column and relieve the nerve pressure, thus restoring energy flow.

Chiropractic physicians treat patients without resorting to drugs or surgery. They may, however, recommend vitamin and mineral supplements or herbs that could help to relieve muscular tension, strengthen the bone and soft tissue of the body, or address certain nutritional deficiencies that may aggravate the patient's condition. They may also recommend an exercise regimen to support the treatment program. In many cases, a chiropractor works in conjunction with a massage therapist, nutritionist, herbalist, or other natural health professional.

Chiropractic has been shown to offer effective relief from a wide range of conditions, including headaches, back and joint pain, respiratory conditions, heart trouble, arthritis, gastrointestinal disorders, menstrual difficulties, and even mental and emotional problems. In some cases, longstanding conditions such as visual disturbances or speech problems also disappear when spinal nerve pressure is relieved through chiropractic.

For many years, the chiropractic profession was under constant attack from mainstream medicine, which viewed chiropractic with extreme skepticism. More recently, however, as more people have grown weary of pharmaceutical drugs and surgery and become interested in natural alternatives, chiropractic has gained a higher profile. Research studies have confirmed the effectiveness of chiropractic for various conditions. In the last decade of the twentieth century, the profession enjoyed increasing recognition and acceptance, resulting in the establishment of chiropractic departments in hospitals and medical clinics.

Today, chiropractic continues to grow and develop, with several techniques being employed that offer variations of the original method, adding new perspectives and dimensions to a profession that is still evolving into a greater understanding of its own potential.

Edgar Cayce frequently recommended chiropractic treatments, sometimes designating a specific practitioner to carry out the chiropractic adjustments. Several readings stress the importance of gentle muscle manipulations along with spinal adjustments. For instance, to the question, "Would a chiropractor help?" in reading 3867-1, Cayce responded: *"Chiropractor would help, but the manipulations with the adjustments will be better."* According to the readings, it is important that muscular relaxation precedes the adjustments of the vertebrae, as explained in reading 1317-1, given for a schoolmaster suffering from anemia: *"The services of an osteopath or a chiropractor . . . where there is used the method of first relaxing the whole of the segment areas, especially in the dorsal and cervical as indicated, and the lumbar and coccyx area; and then adjustments made—not by sudden movements of the segments but a gentle movement, and all made to coordinate."*

In some instances, Cayce advised against chiropractic, recommending instead osteopathy or massage. In other cases, however, the reverse was indicated. In general, chiropractic was recommended when the need for spinal adjustments was predominant, while osteopathy or massage was preferred where there was a primary need for muscular relaxation.

In a letter that Edgar Cayce's stenographer and secretary, Gladys Davis, enclosed with reading 1017-1, she wrote: *"See [attached] letter to Chiropractor with directions for his treatments. Be sure you get a Chiropractor instead of an Osteopath or Naturopath or some other, because it seems that the Chiropractor is especially trained in making that coccyx-lumbar correction referred to in the reading, where the other schools of treating are not."*

In each case, the specific skill and talent of the individual practitioner played the most important role, as shown in the response to the question, "Would you recommend an osteopath?" in reading 3879-1: *"No, neuropath or chiropractor. One, who knows his business. Sometime[s] they don't know their business, you see."*

In his book *A Time to Heal*, chiropractic physician Daniel Redwood addresses the frequently discussed question of whether or not Edgar Cayce favored chiropractic or osteopathy: "One question that often arises with regard to the Cayce readings is whether the principles and practices mentioned there are best represented by contemporary osteopathy or chiropractic. In my judgment, the real answer is neither. The closest analog to the Cayce readings is the osteopathy of the early twentieth century, and practitioners utilizing those methods are now few and far between."

Whether the choice is chiropractic or osteopathy, the guidelines that emerge from the readings are that the gentler manipulations of the muscles and soft tissue were to precede the more forceful adjustments, and that the success of the treatment depended on the proper coordination of both.

In the following section, we will look at the various treatment options offered by osteopathy.

Osteopathy

"Remove all obstructions, and when it is intelligently done, nature will kindly do the rest." These are the words of Dr. Andrew Taylor Still, the founder of osteopathy. Still was born in Jonesboro, Virginia (now known as Jonesville), in 1828. His father was both a Methodist minister and a physician. Young Andrew Still followed in his father's footsteps and became a physician himself. He was also a man of faith, believing that the human body was God's perfect creation and as such held within it the potential for perfect health. Out of frustration with the ineffectiveness of medical treatments of his day and the widespread practice of purging and leeching, Still searched for alternatives, dissecting numerous human corpses and studying bone structure. He spent years developing a healing system that aimed at restoring normal function in the body through the gentle manipulation of tissues and fluids.

Still's theory of osteopathy holds that organ disease has a musculoskeletal component which obstructs the patient's health and that the appropriate manipulation of joints and muscle tissue helps to remove such blockages and to reestablish the proper flow of blood supply, nerve supply, and drainage. The effectiveness of this flow both affects, and is dependent on, the body's nutritional status, which determines the quality of the nutrients available in the blood stream.

This model is highly compatible with the concept of a proper balance between the forces of circulation, assimilation, and elimination that is often stressed in the Cayce readings. If the flow of blood or lymph is impeded, restricting circulation, then the body's ability to assimilate nutrients and eliminate waste will be reduced. At the same time, the nourishing potential of the blood that is circulating in the body depends on the quality of the nutrients that have been assimilated after passing through the organs of digestion and absorption. And without proper elimination, toxic substances accumulate and both circulation and assimilation are severely impeded. Thus, the concept of removing obstructions and restoring the circulation becomes just as important as proper nutrition, especially because both factors synergistically support and affect each other.

Osteopathic treatment was often recommended in the Cayce readings. Reading 1158–31 suggests that *"There is no form of physical mechano-therapy so near in accord with* nature's *measures as correctly given osteopathic adjustments."* A man who wanted to know whether he should go to a chiropractor or an osteopath was told in reading 1415–1 to consult *"Preferably the osteopath; for chiropractic treatment in this particular condition would be rather severe, making too great a strain. For, as has been indicated, these manipulations should be begun* gently . . . *The body should be prepared for the corrections, rather than making the specific adjustments in the beginning."* It was important that there would be *"the massage which goes with correcting along the segments in the cerebrospinal system . . . "* (5391–1)

Dr. Still's method was based on such gentle manipulations and massage, rather than chiropractic's quick, forceful thrusts aimed at realigning vertebrae that might be out of position. Since Andrew Still's and Cayce's time, both osteopathy and chiropractic have evolved, and each discipline has adopted techniques that may not have been part of the original method. For the patient, it is important to find a practitioner with whom one feels comfortable and who is prepared to adjust his or her treatment method to the specific needs of each patient. Reading 5391–1 concluded by suggesting that the questioner find an osteopath, emphasizing that she should *"choose a good one!"*

It is interesting to note that Dr. Andrew Still himself possessed clairvoyant abilities. He was reportedly able to diagnose medical conditions in individuals, even if they were in distant locations. His life's work was not built upon this gift, however. During his lifetime, Dr. Still's unorthodox views and therapeutic measures were severely criticized by his fellow physicians, and he was ostracized by his profession. Undeterred, Still moved forward with his vision of establishing a more effective system of health care. In 1892, he founded the American School of Osteopathy, which is now called the Kirksville College of Osteopathic Medicine.

Today, doctors of osteopathy are the fastest growing segment of health care providers, representing 6 percent of the total U.S. physician population and 8 percent of all military physicians. While in 1982, there were 20,000 osteopathic physicians in practice, this number is expected to quadruple by the year 2020. In the U.S., practitioners of osteopathic medicine are fully licensed physicians, authorized to prescribe medication and perform surgery. However, in addition to having completed the same academic training as their M.D. colleagues, doctors of osteopathy (D.O.s) have received several hundred hours of instruction in the study of the body's musculoskeletal system.

A study published in the November 4, 1999, issue of the *New England Journal of Medicine* found that osteopathic medicine was as effective for low back pain as the standard medical treatment, which includes analgesics and anti-inflammatory medication, but that osteopathy was less expensive and involved less medication for the patient.

Andrew Still passed away in December 1917 at the age of 89. His courage, wisdom, and persistence had paved the way for a drugless, natural system of medicine that continues to serve as a model for holistic practitioners in many disciplines. In Dr. Still's words, *"To find health should be the object of the doctor. Anyone can find disease."*

Therapeutic Massage and Lymphatic Drainage

Dr. Andrew Still's legacy is a constant reminder to the healing professions, as well as to patients, that stagnation of body energies is a major cause of disease. Manipulation to remove obstructions helps to free up energy flow and restore health. Therapeutic massage is an excellent method for doing this, as the therapists' hands work directly with body tissues to release such blockages. In reading 2456-4, Edgar Cayce offered an explanation of the primary reasons an individual should get a massage:

> The "why" of the massage should be considered: Inactivity causes many of those portions along the spine from which impulses are received to the various organs to be lax, or taut, or to allow some to receive greater impulse than others. The massage aids the ganglia to receive impulse[s] from nerve forces as it aids circulation through the various portions of the organism.   2456-4

Inactivity causes stagnation; massage increases circulation, thus reversing the detrimental consequences of inactivity. In therapeutic massage, manual stimulation in the form of kneading, stroking, rolling, wringing, or tapping of the skin and muscle tissue promotes the flow of blood and lymph in the body. In this way, massage helps to flush away toxins and to bring nourishment to the cells via the blood flow. Massage eases tension in the body, soothes the nerves, and promotes rest, relaxation, and healthful sleep. The benefits of therapeutic massage extend beyond the physical into the mental, emotional, and spiritual realms, as it restores a sense of calm, poise, and well-being in the individual.

Hippocrates, the father of Western medicine, believed massage to be an important tool for building and maintaining health. In the twentieth century, distracted by the advent of pharmaceutical drugs and hi-tech health care procedures, mainstream medicine in North America fell out of touch with the benefits of massage. Today's enlightened holistic physicians, however, have rediscovered its wonderful healing potential. In his excellent book *Heal Arthritis: Physically-Mentally-Spiritually*, Dr. William A. McGarey writes: *"We cannot avoid the importance of massage to the body, perhaps as much through a healing touch as through the actual physiological-neurological changes elicited."* Indeed, therapeutic massage is one of the most important health maintenance tools we possess. Today at last, it is gaining greater recognition among health professionals as an adjunct to medical treatment, and as an effective means for the prevention of disease.

A major way in which massage benefits the body is by promoting the optimal function of the lymph system, which is the body's major waste removal mechanism. The lymph system also constitutes an important part of the immune system. Lymph fluid flows along a network of pathways resembling the circulatory system of the blood. In fact, the lymph vessels originate in the small lymph capillaries directly adjacent to the blood capillaries. The lymph acts as a scavenger in the system, picking up waste particles from the cells and facilitating their breakdown and elimination from the body. Viruses and bacteria are also filtered out by the lymph.

The spleen, tonsils, and thymus also form part of the lymphatic system. Their immune-supportive role has often been underestimated, as was evident in the indiscriminate surgical removal of children's tonsils in recent medical history, which is now known to have been based on the inaccurate assumption that the tonsils were superfluous body parts. We know today that the tonsils are interceptors of bacteria entering the throat—a primary site of the body's immunological activity against disease.

A major function of the lymphatics is to return serum proteins that normally seep out of the blood capillaries, to the blood. The lymph also carries nutrients to the cells, and removes waste products and foreign particles. This cellular waste material is transported along the lymphatic vessels to special filtering stations called lymph nodes, which filter out and destroy any debris, viruses, or bacteria. The freshly cleaned lymph fluid then continues to travel along the lymphatic pathways on to the heart.

Keeping the lymph flowing freely through the body is crucial to maintaining good health. Of key importance is the fact that the lymphatic system depends largely on muscular contraction to move the lymph along its pathways. Some continuous lymph flow is ensured by the peristaltic action of the intestine, as well as by the lungs and diaphragm during breathing. Lymph flow from the extremities, however, is almost entirely dependent on muscle movement or on manipulation, such as massage.

With today's sedentary lifestyles, muscles often don't get enough exercise to adequately stimulate efficient lymph flow. This, combined with poor dietary habits and environmental pollution, places an excessive burden on the lymph system. The result is often lymphatic congestion, indicated by enlargement, inflammation, and hardening of the lymph nodes, lymphatic vessels, and organs. Ultimately, the immune response is lowered, making us more susceptible not only to short-term illnesses and infections, but also to chronic degenerative disease.

By stimulating the flow of lymph and improving drainage from the tissues and lymphatic pathways, therapeutic massage helps to detoxify the body, strengthen the immune system, and prevent chronic degenerative conditions.

Some massage therapists and naturopathic physicians are trained in a special technique called Manual Lymph Drainage (MLD), which applies light strokes to the skin to effect a pumping action in the lymphatic vessels. MLD was designed by the physical therapists Emil and

Astrid Vodder in France in the 1930s. MLD is very popular in Europe, where it is part of the standard therapy in the treatment of cellulite, a condition mostly affecting women in which unsightly lumps of fat form on the thighs, hips, and buttocks. But the concept underlying MLD goes back thousands of years. In the millennia–old Indian medical system of Ayurveda, maintenance of the lymphatics is given high priority. A healthy flow of lymph is associated with the attributes of good nourishment and articulation of joints, viscosity, and sexual stamina, and with virtues such as fortitude, patience, and solidarity.

In Ayurveda, the lymphatic system is governed by the *Kapha*, or mucus–carrying energies. For the symptoms of lymphatic congestion, and as part of its daily health–regimen, Ayurveda prescribes a whole–body massage. For those without access to a massage therapist, Ayurveda recommends a self–massage to those parts of the body which are easily accessible.

The condition of lymph in the body also influences psychological well–being, according to Harish Johari, author of the book *Ancient Indian Massage*. He says that lymph fluid contains a relatively large amount of the amino acid tryptophan, which the body converts to serotonin. Symptoms of serotonin depletion, such as anxiety and irritability, appear to be relieved by lymphatic massage, indicating a possible increase of serotonin levels. Johari postulates that the hormone melatonin, also derived from tryptophan, is augmented by lymphatic stimulation, and may be responsible for the pleasant, calming effects of massage. He further suggests that lymph may be the body's own natural anti–histamine, since it also contains high levels of histaminase, the enzyme which breaks down histamine, the major chemical involved in the body's allergic response.

The Lymph System and Castor Oil Packs. The Cayce readings also provide an unusual perspective on lymphatic function, placing special importance on the Peyer's patches, which are tiny patches of lymphatic tissue in the mucosal surface of the small intestine. According to Cayce, the Peyer's patches produce a substance which facilitates electrical contact between the autonomous and the cerebrospinal nervous systems when it reaches those areas via the bloodstream. Dr. William A. McGarey, who has clinically worked with castor oil packs and other suggestions from the Cayce readings for several decades, understands Cayce to say that the health of the entire nervous system is, to an extent, maintained through the substances produced by the Peyer's patches when they are in good health. Although these patches were discovered in 1677, it is only recently that medical science has begun to recognize that they constitute part of the immune system. Cayce suggested that the use of castor oil packs on the body can strengthen the Peyer's patches and have a direct effect on the autonomic nervous system.

In following Cayce's suggestion throughout the years of his medical career, Dr. McGarey has found that the application of warm castor oil packs over different parts of the body stimulates the lymphatics and brings about a degree of healing by stimulating the immune response. In keeping with Cayce's recommendations, particular attention is paid to the abdominal area, where a large concentration of lymph nodes is located.

Current research confirms the efficacy of castor oils packs in improving immune response. A double-blind study, described by Harvey Grady in a report entitled *Immunomodulation through Castor Oil Packs* published in *The Journal of Naturopathic Medicine* (Vol. 7, No. 1) examined lymphocyte values of thirty-six healthy subjects before and after topical castor oil application. This study identified castor oil as an antitoxin, and as having an impact on the lymphatic system, enhancing immunological function. The study found that castor oil pack therapy of a minimal two-hour duration produced an increase in the number of T-11 cells within a twenty-four-hour period following treatment, with a concomitant increase in the number of total lymphocytes. This T-11 cell increase represents a general boost in the body's specific defense status, since lymphocytes actively defend the health of the body by forming antibodies against pathogens and their toxins. T-cells identify and kill viruses, fungi, bacteria, and cancer cells.

Dr. McGarey has summarized his extensive experiences related to castor oil and its effects on the lymphatic and immune systems in a fascinating book, *The Oil That Heals*. The following instructions for preparing castor oil packs at home are excerpted from this book:

"Prepare a flannel cloth which is two or three thicknesses when folded and which measures about eight inches in width and ten to twelve inches in length after it is folded. This is the size needed for abdominal application—other areas may need a different size pack, as seems applicable. Pour castor oil into a pan and soak the cloth in the oil. Wring out the cloth so that it is wet but not drippy with the castor oil (or simply pour castor oil onto the pack so it is soaked). Apply the cloth to the area which needs treatment. Most often, the pack should be placed so it covers the area of the liver.

"Protection against soiling bed clothing can be made by putting a plastic sheet underneath the body. Then a plastic covering should be applied over the soaked flannel cloth. On top of the plastic place a heating pad and turn it up to "medium" to begin, then to "high" if the body tolerates it. It helps to wrap a large towel around the body to hold the pack snugly in place, using large safety pins on the towel. The pack should remain in place between an hour to an hour and a half.

"The skin can be cleansed afterwards, if desired, by using water which is prepared as follows: to a quart of water, add two teaspoons baking soda. Use this to cleanse the abdomen. Keep the flannel pack wrapped in plastic for future use. It need not be discarded after one application, but can usually be used many times."

Note: Always use a high–quality, cold–pressed castor oil, available in health food stores or from manufacturers and retailers of Cayce–recommended products.

Massage Oils.   Therapeutic massage almost always includes the use of oils, such as peanut, almond, grapeseed, sesame, coconut, or olive oil. However, many other types of oil, singly or in combination, may be used. Olive oil is also frequently a constituent of the massage oil formulations found in the Cayce readings, which suggest that it is a "food" for the soft tissues. Thus, while massage oil functions as a lubricant, it also nourishes the skin and underlying tissues. In the Cayce readings, olive oil is often recommended in combination with peanut oil, which is said to be a remedy and a preventive medicine for arthritic conditions. Reading 1158–31 states, *Those who would take a peanut oil rub each week need never fear arthritis.* Many massage therapists who regularly use peanut oil discover that the oil not only benefits patients who suffer from arthritis, but that it also effectively prevents the development of arthritis in the therapists' hands. The quality of the oil used in massage is important because the oils are readily absorbed through the skin. Only mechanically extracted, unrefined oils should be used. Commercial oils that have been extracted with the use of chemicals and that are highly refined, bleached, and deodorized are best avoided.

The Cayce readings provide the following formula for a massage oil mixture that is excellent for stimulating superficial circulation and beautifying the skin: Mix together 6 oz. peanut oil, 2 oz. olive oil, 2 oz. natural rosewater, and 1 tsp. dissolved lanolin, and shake well. This formula is easy to prepare, but it is best made in small quantities, as natural rosewater spoils easily and, when combined with oils, promotes rancidity. Commercial versions of this formula are available from manufacturers of Cayce-recommended products.

A study conducted at the University College of Medical Sciences in Delhi, India, found that oil massage promotes growth in infants and helps the babies to sleep better. Over a period of four weeks, the infants, who were approximately six weeks old, received an oil massage daily for a total of ten minutes. In comparison to the control group that did not receive a massage, the infants who received the oil massage had greater weight, body length, head circumference, and girth of arm and leg.

Several readings that Edgar Cayce gave for infants included recommendations for a gentle massage along the spine. Often this massage was to be done after a bath given in the evenings before the child fell asleep. This was said to relax and help to coordinate the nervous and glandular systems. Peanut oil or cocoa butter were often recommended as massage lubricants. In reading 928-1, Cayce gave the following suggestions for a three-week-old girl suffering from colic: *"It would be well that the spine, especially over the upper dorsal (or from the neck to the middle or lower portion of the waist), be massaged with cocoa butter. This massaging should be very gentle, to be sure, and with the hands warm; as well as the coca butter being warm (though not hot) as it is massaged. Do this once or twice a day."*

It is interesting to note that in Ayurvedic massage, massage oils are always "cured" by being heated and should be at, or slightly above, body temperature when applied.

Massage Techniques.   There are several different methods that
massage therapists use to work on an individual. In the western hemi-
sphere, Swedish massage is the most commonly practiced technique. It
was developed as a medical treatment in Sweden in the mid–1800s and
was introduced to North America less than half a century later. It is,
however, based on techniques first practiced in ancient China about
2700 B.C. Swedish massage emphasizes basic strokes of the soft tissue,
working toward the heart. Swedish massage also incorporates techniques such as kneading, tapping, and rolling.

Dr. Harold Reilly (see Introduction for details), the founder of the
Cayce/Reilly School of Massotherapy, was trained in Swedish massage.
Many of Reilly's massage concepts were based on Swedish massage, but
his lifelong investigation into the material from the Cayce readings and
many other healing modalities led him to develop variations of the
original method. Reilly had extensive knowledge of osteopathy, chiropractic, and physical therapy, and thus had the ideal background for
extrapolating the relevant recommendations from the readings that
made reference to such techniques. As mentioned in the Introduction,
the Cayce readings referred many individuals to Harold Reilly, despite
the fact that he and Edgar Cayce had never met or heard of each other
prior to these referrals. Special highlights of the Cayce/Reilly massage
include a technique called "nerve compression," which aims to normalize the circulation of nerve forces. There is also an emphasis on joint
mobilization, stretches, and special range–of–motion movements that
help to lubricate the joints by promoting the release of synovial fluid.
The Cayce–recommended spinal massage, aimed at coordinating the
central nervous system with the autonomic nervous system, also forms
part of this technique, which continues to be taught and practiced at
the Cayce/Reilly School of Massotherapy in Virginia Beach, Virginia.
Details of the Cayce/Reilly technique, which can be adapted for use at
home with family and friends, are explained in Harold Reilly's *The Edgar
Cayce Handbook for Health Through Drugless Therapy*.

Oriental Massage and Acupressure.   In Oriental medical philosophy, the major internal organs are represented by what might be explained as "energy zones" in different areas of the body. A vital force referred to as *chi* traverses these fields, flowing along the meridian lines, which are related to the different internal organs. In a healthy body, the flow of *chi* is even and uninterrupted, resulting in a perfect balance of the expansive and contractive forces of yin and yang. Where the flow of *chi* is excessive or restricted, an imbalance is created that eventually manifests in symptoms of disease.

For instance, Chinese medicine teaches that the lumbar region is the "residence of the kidneys," but this refers to more than their physiological function. The kidney energy also rules the urogenital tract and glandular activities, and it is closely related to the central nervous system, as well as the respiratory and digestive systems. Even the bones are considered to be controlled by the kidneys. A deficiency of kidney energy can produce symptoms such as lower back pain which intensifies with stress, weak knees, and general fatigue. Depression and insomnia, along with impotence or low sperm count in men, and menstrual irregularities, infertility, or lack of sexual response in women, are additional indications of reduced kidney energy. Massage, as well as acupressure, can help to correct such imbalances by either stimulating or toning down the flow of *chi* along the respective meridians.

The Japanese use a technique called *shiatsu*, composed of *shi*—finger, and *atsu*—pressure. Shiatsu employs finger pressure, either from the finger tips or from the knuckles, to balance meridian energies. Sometimes, the pressure is applied with the elbow or base of the palm. Shiatsu therapists also use rotating, shaking, pinching, and rolling movements. A skilled shiatsu therapist is able to identify energy imbalances in the body by placing a hand on the client's abdomen and sensing and observing the *chi* flowing through the *hara*—the abdominal area. "Hara diagnosis," along with other diagnostic methods such as pulse diagnosis, enables the practitioner to gain a comprehensive understanding of a person's specific treatment needs. Shiatsu helps to relieve tension in the body, improve the flow of blood and lymph, promote digestion and assimilation, lessen pain, and reduce movement restrictions. It also indirectly treats specific organ "deficiencies" or imbalances.

Like Swedish massage and other methods of therapeutic manipulation, shiatsu aims at removing obstructions and restoring energy flow throughout the body. The specific techniques may differ, but their ultimate goal is the same: to awaken the body's innate healing force and allow it to recreate health on the physical, mental, emotional, and spiritual levels.

Body Electronics. Most therapists who have worked with massage or other methods of therapeutic manipulation have occasionally witnessed a strong emotional response from an individual undergoing treatment. The person may suddenly begin to laugh hysterically or cry uncontrollably. They may simultaneously remember traumatic events in their life that had been suppressed or forgotten. Apparently the release of physical energy, facilitated by the massage or finger pressure, results in a release of stored memories, which bring to the surface the emotions that had been suppressed along with those memories. Many holistic practitioners are convinced that physical aches and pains often pinpoint the locations in the body where suppressed emotions are stored. The Cayce readings acknowledge that negative emotions can become detrimental to the health of the physical body. Reading 849-75 says: " . . . *when there is any anger, it prepares the system so that it blocks the flow of the circulation to the eliminating channels,*" while reading 2189-3 explains: " . . . *depressions, anger, wrath, sorrow, and such, make for poisons in the digestive system, causing an activity of an unnatural or abnormal manner through same.*"

The late Dr. John Whitman Ray (1934–2001), a naturopathic physician, psychologist, mathematician, and *Pax Mundi* award recipient, was the founder of Body Electronics, a technique that uses sustained finger pressure to release suppressed memory and trauma from body tissues. Over many years of working with naturopathic healing techniques, Ray discovered that in the human body, tissue calcifications—crystals, as he called them—function in ways similar to computer chips, or microchips, that hold encoded information. As such, a body "crystal" can be likened to an "organic computer chip" full of stored memories, most often suppressed beneath conscious awareness. Through the application of sustained finger pressure directly on the part of the body where the calcification is located, it is possible to dissolve the crystal. In Body Electronics, this process is appropriately referred to as "point-holding."

As the crystal is gradually being broken down with sustained pressure—for minutes and even hours at a time—the person who is undergoing point–holding mentally reexperiences the events and accompanying emotional reactions that, because they had not been fully dealt with, had become locked into the calcified body tissues. Simultaneously, the individual is being encouraged, in an accepting and supportive environment, to reexperience these emotions with full awareness and to subsequently release them with unconditional love and complete forgiveness for all persons who may have contributed to the pain that was originally suppressed and thus encoded into the crystal. Once these emotions are lovingly and willingly reexperienced, the person who is the subject of such a point–holding session will consecutively experience feelings such as numbness, pain, heat or cold, and "electrical" jolts, or throbbing. John Ray referred to this as the experience of the "burning, searing fire" of the kundalini force that is breaking down the crystal and cleansing the body of accumulated calcifications. When this happens, the person holding the points may often feel extreme heat at the point of the finger, thumb, or elbow with which the pressure is being applied. It is essential, at that point, that the pressure be sustained until the heat subsides, indicating that the crystal has broken down completely.

John Ray taught that such crystals are more easily dissolved when the body is nutritionally prepared with "nutrient saturation," meaning that all necessary nutrients are available to the tissues in optimal amounts. Therefore, a sound nutrition program, emphasizing natural whole foods, food–based supplements, and enzymes, are an important aspect of Body Electronics. Holistic health professionals, whether they are chiropractors, osteopaths, massage therapists, or practitioners of other disciplines, will agree that those who eat a whole foods diet and lead a lifestyle that is in accordance with nature respond better to therapeutic manipulation than those whose diets are less than optimal. No aspect of health must be neglected if a therapy is to produce the desired results. As Cayce reading 1945–1 says: " . . . *the diet as well as the mental attitude of the body towards creative or spiritual influences in its life* must *be a part of those applications for beneficial conditions."*

Through Body Electronics, many people have successfully released long–suppressed feelings of fear, anger, pain, and resistance and have simultaneously overcome the accompanying physical blockages that produced symptoms ranging from mild discomfort to serious physical disabilities and deformities. What brings such healing about? A change in the consciousness of the affected cells of the body as destructive feelings and emotions are released and replaced with love and forgive-ness. In *Heal Arthritis: Physically-Mentally-Spiritually,* Dr. William A. McGarey writes: *"For healing to occur, a change in consciousness must come about—in other words, a divine happening must occur within the consciousness of the cells and at-oms of the body itself."*

The aim of Body Electronics is not only to help free the individual of long–held and locked–in destructive emotions and physical symptoms, but also to enable them to live fully in the present and to respond to each event in their life with unconditional love, rather than react from unconsciously held patterns of conduct. John Ray taught that one must learn to release all patterns of resistances such as old grudges and hard feelings with unconditional love and unconditional forgiveness. He said that the faults we see in others which attract our attention should be an immediate signal to go inside and search for the error in our thinking.

The Cayce readings echo these sentiments: *"To be sure, attitudes oft influ-ence the physical conditions of the body. No one can hate his neighbor and not have stomach or liver trouble. No one can be jealous and allow the anger of same and not have upset digestion or heart disorder."* (4021-1) And *"Do not find fault. For he that finds fault with his brother is guilty already of the same."* (270-34)

Therapeutic Touch. Considering the degree of skepticism with which mainstream medicine views most alternative healing approaches, it is nearly miraculous that an esoteric technique such as Therapeutic Touch is being taught and practiced in many hospitals and medical schools across North America. Therapeutic Touch was developed in the early 1970s by Dolores Krieger, Ph.D., R.N. It draws its origins in the ancient religious practice of laying on of hands, but it also incorporates other techniques, such as visualization, prayer, and aura therapy. Pri-marily it involves the subtle manipulation and balancing of a person's energy field, often referred to as the "aura."

A practitioner of Therapeutic Touch typically uses some techniques to become quietly centered prior to beginning a treatment, asking to be the vehicle through which the Holy Spirit of God might flow and help to heal the patient. This process also connects the practitioner to the patient on an energetic level. Next, the practitioner, who might be a nurse, a doctor, or other therapist, holds his or her hands with palms down about one to three inches from the patient's body, and then moves them along the person's energy field, sensing any irregularities which might be experienced as heat, cold, or a change in vibration. Any areas of stagnation or imbalance in the body will be identified by such ir-regularities. With continued focused intent, the practitioner then uses a number of motions to balance the patient's energy, sometimes perform-ing stroking or sweeping movements of the hands. Some Therapeutic Touch practitioners include the physical laying on of hands in their treatment protocol.

Clinical studies have confirmed the clinical experience of thousands of patients who say they have been benefited by Therapeutic Touch. The technique has been shown to relieve pain, and reduce fever and inflammation, as well as stress and anxiety. Physiologically measurable changes in enzyme activity and hemoglobin levels, along with acceler-ated wound healing, have also been observed.

Therapeutic Touch is a simple yet powerful healing technique. Its ability to ease problems associated with autonomic nervous system dysfunc-tion—a widespread condition in today's hectic world—makes it the per-fect antidote to modern ills. From the perspective of the Cayce readings, the amazing healing effects of Therapeutic Touch are readily explained: *"It is true then that the mind may heal entirely by the spoken word, by the laying on of hands, dependent upon the consciousness of the motivative forces in the indi-vidual body."* (262–83) The rapid integration of the Therapeutic Touch tech-nique into mainstream medicine is a powerful tribute to this statement.

Hydrotherapy. Many people underestimate just how significant water is for the health of the body—inside and out. Water is the most abundant substance in nature. About three-fourths of the earth's surface is covered with water. The human body consists of over 60 percent water.

Water is ubiquitous in most industrialized countries, and in those parts of the world, few people go thirsty for long before they can get themselves a drink. It is difficult to imagine, therefore, that dehydration may be at the root of many of our modern ills. But Dr. F. Batmanghelidj, author of *Your Body's Many Cries for Water*, believes that most people are chronically dehydrated without being aware of the problem. By restoring adequate water intake in his patients, he has helped them overcome numerous conditions including allergies, back pain, high blood pressure, asthma, chronic fatigue syndrome, ulcers, and high cholesterol levels. The Cayce readings concur with Batmanghelidj, suggesting that *"The body should keep the whole system, inside and out, thoroughly cleansed with water, drinking water as medicine, or in . . . regular intervals and drinking sufficient."* (4771-1)

In the body, water is required for digestion and the elimination of toxins and waste products. We depend on water to deliver nutrients to the cells, and for the circulation of blood, lymph, and interstitial fluids. Water is needed for the regulation of body temperature, as well as for the maintenance of electrolyte and osmotic pressure balance. Without water intake, we cannot survive for more than a few days. Most health experts agree that the optimal water intake per person per day is between six and ten eight-ounce glasses, depending on body weight, activity level, diet, and environmental conditions. The Cayce readings suggest to *"drink plenty of water through the day, at least six to eight tumblers full."* (2341-1) It is best to sip the water in small amounts throughout the day, ideally between meals. *"Do not drink water with meals. Take the water between the [meal] periods . . . "* (5647-1) Drinking excessive amounts of water with meals dilutes the digestive juices, thus reducing the ability to digest and assimilate foods properly. If sufficient water is taken between meals, the body won't be as thirsty at meal time.

It is important to realize that not all liquids count as water when adding up one's daily intake. Cola drinks and soda pops, with their high sugar content, increase the need for pure water. Coffee and black tea are water robbers, since they have a diuretic effect. It is better to drink unsweetened herbal teas instead. As a thirst-quencher and detoxifier, however, nothing works better than water itself.

Water heals both from the inside out and from the outside in. The health and appearance of our skin depends on adequate internal water intake. And water treatments applied externally to the skin can promote healing of a diseased organ or muscle tissue.

Sebastian Kneipp, a nineteenth–century Bavarian priest, utilized water compresses, wraps, baths, and steam treatments to heal thousands of ill people. Now recognized worldwide as one of the founders of naturopathy, Kneipp himself provided the best example of the miraculous healing powers of water. In his early twenties, weakened by working long hours in a damp weaving room to support his studies for the priesthood, Kneipp contracted tuberculosis. He grew so ill that his physicians gave up hope that he would ever recover.

An avid reader, even on his deathbed, Kneipp came across a book that was a compilation of Johann Sigmund Hahn's *Lectures on the Wonderful Healing Powers of Fresh Water*. Since he lacked the funds to pay for further medical help, Kneipp began to work on himself with the cold–water treatments outlined in the book. With determination and persistence he succeeded, achieving a complete recovery several months later.

After he entered the priesthood in 1852, Kneipp began to treat his parishioners with the water therapy that had helped him to regain health. Word of his miraculous cures spread quickly, and he began to attract patients from all over the world. In Europe today, Kneipp's name is synonymous with hydrotherapy, and his teachings continue to influence modern naturopathy worldwide.

Although diet and herbs were part of Kneipp's overall health regimen, his main focus consisted of applying cold water by various means to the patient's body. One of his favorite recommendations was walking barefoot in the dewy morning grass, or in freshly fallen snow. He believed that this would stimulate circulation and strengthen resistance to illness. In one of his writings, Kneipp explains: *"Those who go barefoot never suffer from cold feet, which is the result of poorness of blood and too little of it . . . I recommend going barefoot not only as a relief, but as protection against many diseases peculiar to those who lead a sedentary life in which the brain has too much to do and the body little."* Although this was written over a hundred years ago (in 1897), hardly anyone can argue that the majority of the population today falls into this category. The Cayce readings agree on the importance of balancing mental activity with physical activity outdoors. For instance, reading 341–31 states: *"Take more outdoor exercise . . . that brings into play the muscular forces of the body. It isn't that the mental should be numbed, or should be cut off from their operations or their activities—but make for a more evenly, more perfectly balanced body—physical and mental."*

Another version of Kneipp's barefoot walk is treading in cold water. Cold water wading basins are found along numerous hiking paths in the mountainous regions of southern Bavaria, where the traveler can observe hikers remove their shoes and socks, take an invigorating water walk, and then continue on their way refreshed and energized. Others take an "elbow bath," which consists of immersing the lower arms up to the elbows in a cold water basin.

Kneipp Therapy At Home. Although nothing can totally simulate the energizing effect of fresh mountain spring water, it is fairly easy to try some of the water treatments at home. If you have access to dewy field or meadows, take off your shoes and go for a walk or run. An inflatable kiddie pool in the backyard is great for water wading. Or try it in your bathtub, being sure to avoid slipping.

Sebastian Kneipp also used a watering can or hose to apply a gush of cold water to a specific part of the body, for instance the thigh or knee. This increases circulation to the area and promotes healing. Also effective for this purpose are wraps, in which a cloth is saturated with cold water and then wrapped around the torso, leg, or arm.

Conditions which have successfully responded to Kneipp therapy include anemia, arthritis, cardiovascular problems, digestive disturbances, migraine headaches, skin problems, and rheumatism. Repetition and persistence are essential if a long-lasting effect is to be achieved.

An excellent overall water treatment that can be incorporated into most people's daily schedule is rinsing off the body with cold water after a warm bath or shower. Simply turn on the cold water and remain there for as long as you can stand it, or move in and out of the cold stream. The first few moments might feel uncomfortable but, with practice, you will soon get used to it and come to appreciate the energizing, refreshing effect of finishing your shower or bath with a cold water gush.

A more elaborate version of this procedure is alternating hot and cold showers. Begin with warm water, then cold, then increase the temperature of the warm water to maximum comfort levels. Always finish with cold water.

Therapeutic footbaths have many useful applications. Have you noticed that it is difficult to fall asleep when your feet are cold? One of the best remedies for this annoying problem, which keeps numerous people awake at night, especially during the winter season, is a cold, or alternating hot–and–cold footbath at bedtime. This draws stagnant energy from the upper part of the body, balances circulation, and warms the feet quickly. After the footbath, slip on a pair of socks, and crawl under the covers. You won't be waiting long for the sandman to come!

Water in our environment can also influence our health and psychological well–being in many different ways. Certain water veins below the earth's surface are said to make us ill in the same way that low-frequency electrical currents do. But the regions surrounding lakes and oceans are favorite destinations for relaxation and recreational pursuits. Just being near them often makes us feel better and happier. Apart from physiologically measurable results, such as the health–promoting effect of beneficial mineral particles in ocean air, there appear to be definite psychological and spiritual influences that are felt in the presence of water.

When Edgar Cayce was searching for a suitable location to establish a research organization and to further develop his activities, his own psychic counsel advised him to seek out the town of Virginia Beach, situated by the Atlantic Ocean, because proximity to a large body of water was said to be beneficial for the progression of his psychic work. Thus, it was in Virginia Beach that the Association for Research and Enlightenment was founded in 1931. The work of the organization continues to this day.

Throughout the ages, there has been a perceived link between water and spirit. Some waters, such as those from a spring in Lourdes, France, are credited with having supernatural healing powers. "Holy water" in the Catholic faith is used to spiritually purify and bless people and places. In baptism, water is used as a symbol of initiation.

Bath Therapy. Various forms of bathing—full baths, sitz baths, other partial baths, and fume baths—also form part of the water treatments that were recommended in the Cayce readings. These types of baths are also extensively applied in European health care facilities as part of the standard hydrotherapy regimen. Baths help to increase circulation, remove toxins from the body via the skin, and encourage muscular relaxation. Both hot and cold baths serve to increase circulation, but they do so in different ways. Hot baths are most effective to help sweat out toxins, while cold baths help to relieve congestion and invigorate the body. Warm baths have the greatest relaxing effect. Researchers at Kagoshima University in Japan have found that warm baths improve exercise endurance in the elderly. Some of the subjects in the small study had a heart condition, while others did not, but a ten-minute bath in 106–degree Fahrenheit water improved exercise capacity for both groups. Bath regimens that utilize extreme temperatures (hot or cold), however, should only be done under the guidance and supervision of a qualified health professional, due to their strong effects on the cardiovascular system.

Several Cayce readings recommend the addition of Epsom salts to bath water, especially for individuals suffering from arthritic conditions. Epsom salts help to draw toxins from the body, as Cayce acknowledges in reading 2–8: *"Will be well . . . to give those of the baths as will eliminate— especially in those of the Epsom baths, or the fume baths from same."* And reading 1811–1, given for a fifty–year–old woman, suggests: *"Also about once a week there would be the Epsom Salts Bath; not too strong but such that the body would lie in same . . . for at least twenty to thirty minutes; more as the body is able. Use about ten to twelve and a half pounds of Epsom Salts to fifty gallons of water, as warm as the body may well stand."* In some cases, it was suggested that such baths be followed by a massage or rub. Epsom salts were also recommended for use in packs, dissolved in just enough water to saturate a bath towel.

Where baths were to be used for relaxation purposes, the readings recommended the addition of oil of balsam or pine.

Colonic Irrigations. The Cayce readings consistently emphasize the importance of keeping the colon clean—through adequate fiber and water intake, sufficient exercise, and colonic irrigation. The colon is the last collecting station in the passage that food takes through the body. Maintaining regular bowel function is important for colon health, as any fecal matter that remains in the colon can dry out and adhere to the colon walls, which obstructs the colon and slows down the absorption of nutrients. When the colon is thus impacted, it becomes difficult for the beneficial bacteria that are normally present in the colon to survive. Unhealthy bacteria flourish instead, producing toxic by-products. Bowel toxicity has been associated with many health conditions, including arthritis, allergies, headaches, sinus congestion, and skin conditions.

Regular colonic irrigations help to flush out encrusted fecal matter, toxins, and other impurities, resulting in greater energy and better overall health. Cayce reading 440-2 suggests that " . . . every one—*everybody— should take an internal bath occasionally, as well as an external one. They would all be better off if they would!*" In the readings, colonics were recommended for many conditions, including arthritis, asthma, dermatitis, epilepsy, migraine headaches, and high blood pressure.

In a professional colonic, two tubes are inserted into the rectum through a speculum. The pure, lukewarm water is flushed in through one tube, and water and loosened fecal matter and impurities are flushed out through the other. During the process, the colon therapist performs a gentle massage of the client's abdomen, which encourages the flow of water and the cleansing process. A colonic irrigation is deeper than an enema. In fact, Cayce reading 3570-1 claims that *"One colonic irrigation will be worth about four to six enemas."*

Whether we drink our water, bathe in it, or use it to flush out the colon, it is important to make sure that the water is adequately purified. The water that is pumped into our homes from treatment facilities is a far cry from the *aqua pura* that nature created. Most often it has been treated with chlorine, an immuno-suppressant and carcinogenic chemical, and it also delivers numerous inorganic chemicals, toxic metals, and other impurities.

The ideal water is mountain spring water, naturally filtered and mineralized by rocks and gravel, energized by sunlight, and oxygenated by clean air. Unfortunately, this type of water is available to very few in today's world. Most of us must rely on the option of purchasing bottled water, or that of using some type of water purifier or distiller.

Distilled water is preferred by some because the process of distillation guarantees a high degree of purity. On the other hand, it also removes most trace minerals. Some health professionals believe that the long-term consumption of distilled water can lead to a deficiency in important minerals. Others argue that this can easily be prevented or remedied by taking a natural mineral supplement, such as kelp or other seaweeds. The fact remains that pure, mineral–rich spring water is the type of water that nature intended us to drink. Cayce reading 1152–8 echoes this sentiment: *"Fresh spring water or tap water would be preferable to distilled water."* It's important to bear in mind that the tap water that might have been available to the woman for whom the reading was given in 1939 would likely have been of better quality than most tap water is today.

Therapeutic manipulation—whether through chiropractic, osteopathy, massage, or hydrotherapy—represents the simplest, most natural, yet also most effective method of helping others, and ourselves, to gain greater health. As reading 823–1 says: " . . . *the laying on of hands, and the prayers of those that have found patience, may save many from the turmoils and strifes of a dis-ease in a material body."*

Exercise and Rest:
Getting the Balance Right

Exercise in the open and rest would be better than all medicinal properties.
Edgar Cayce reading 4654-1

EVERYWHERE IN NATURE, we can observe a continuous interplay of motion and stillness, activity and inactivity, outward expression and inward receptivity—the yin and yang of Eastern philosophy. Our physical bodies, too, need alternate periods of movement and rest to stay healthy and balanced. Because our modern and often sedentary lifestyles require too little physical activity of us in terms of our everyday living, we need to make an intentional effort to increase that activity through exercise.

We have seen in the previous chapter how the manipulation of body tissues through various forms of massage can help, from the outside in, to remove energy blocks and metabolic waste and stimulate the circulation of blood and lymph. Exercise is a means of achieving similar results through activity from the inside out. Some of the best methods of physical therapy combine manipulation with movement therapy, or passive exercise with active exercise.

Edgar Cayce often stressed the importance of physical exercise, saying in one reading that *"The body should exercise sufficiently to at times be physically tired."* (5718-1) Evidently, the tendency of humans to overexercise the mind but underexercise the body was as prevalent in Cayce's days as it is today.

In recent years, however, scientific research has shown that the mind, in turn, benefits from physical exercise. A preliminary study conducted in 2001 at the University of Illinois in Urbana–Champaign demonstrated that thirty minutes of moderately heavy to heavy running on a treadmill could improve the thinking ability of a group of young men and women. Following the exercise, the speed of the decision–making process was increased in the test subjects, and the answers that respondents provided to test questions also proved more accurate. Also in 2001, researchers at Nihon Fukushi University in Handa, Japan, found that individuals consistently scored higher on intellectual tests after embarking on a running program. The reason this happens is likely improved blood flow in brain tissue and an increase in oxygen intake, both of which translate into improved circulation.

It is interesting to note that when the joggers stopped their training, the improvements diminished, suggesting that ongoing exercise is required to maintain the benefits. The Cayce readings also emphasize that consistency is key to success in any exercise program. Reading 308-13 says: " . . . *regular exercise would be helpful, but don't start this and then do it for a day and then skip two or three days and then try it again; either do it regularly or don't begin . . .* "

Regular exercise has been shown to boost older people's mood, but indeed, to reap the benefits of an exercise program one must commit to keeping it up. This was demonstrated in a study reported in the March 15, 2001, issue of the *American Journal of Epidemiology* which showed that older adults who exercised regularly for a while but later stopped were more likely to develop depression than those who had kept up their physical activity.

The influence of physical activity on overall health is so great that a new set of dietary guidelines issued by the U.S. federal government in May 2000 includes a recommendation for exercise. Exercise is known to improve cardiovascular health. It can thus help to prevent heart disease, America's number–one killer disease. A study conducted at the University of Pisa in Italy showed that exercise keeps the lining of the arteries young, and this may be one of the reasons for the heart–protective effects of exercise. However, regular exercise may also significantly reduce the risk of cancer. Researchers from the Cooper Institute in Dallas, Texas, found that men who were considered to be "unfit" based on treadmill tests were 80 percent more likely to die of cancer than fit men were. In another study done at the University College Medical School in London, U.K., men who vigorously exercised two or more times per week had a 24 percent reduction in cancer risk.

From a holistic perspective, exercise can help to prevent illness by improving circulation of blood and lymph, which promotes cellular detoxification and nourishment. Exercise also gets us sweating, and this may in itself provide a health boost by helping to fight infections, according to a report published in the December 2001 issue of journal *Nature Immunology*. *Dermicidin*, an antimicrobial agent manufactured in the body's sweat glands, secreted into the sweat, and transported to the surface of the skin, is responsible for this action. *Dermicidin* was found to be effective against many different types of bacteria, including E. coli, S. aureus, and Candida albicans. Sweating can also help to remove toxins from the body. The Cayce readings recommend sweating, most often in the form of sweat baths, but also the type of sweating that results from exercise, as suggested in reading 567–5: *"Keep the physical exercises; not strenuous, but consistent, so that the body—whether in walking, in the setting-up exercise, no matter how cold it may be outside—gets up a good sweat; and we will have a better coordination throughout the system."*

This reading also points out that when it comes to exercising, consistency is more important than excessive strain. This is, in fact, what modern health experts are telling consumers. A study reported in the March 29, 2001, issue of the journal *Nature* shows that those who engaged in regular moderate exercise such as walking, biking, or gardening, demonstrated the highest overall physical activity levels compared with those who undertook shorter bouts of intense activity. According to the researchers, such regular moderate exercise may also burn more calories.

Walk for Your Life

Cayce's advice that *"Walking is the best exercise!"* (715–1), repeated in quite a few readings, appears once again to be substantiated by modern research. A study done at Harvard Medical School in Boston, Massachusetts, found that walking decreases women's risk of heart disease. The length of time spent walking each day was a more important determiner of cardiovascular health than walking speed. Among the test subjects, who were all women aged forty–five and older, those who regularly walked an hour or more each day had about half the heart disease risk of those who walked less than an hour. This study was made public in the spring of 2000. In 1943, Cayce had told a thirty–two–year–old woman: *"Walking is the best exercise, but don't take this spasmodically. Have a regular time and do it, rain or shine!"* (1968–9)

Another study, published in the June 14, 2000, issue of *The Journal of the American Medical Association*, showed that regular, moderate exercise such as walking can cut women's risk of stroke. This was true even if the women started walking at an older age, which proves that it is never too late for a change to a healthier lifestyle. Walking has also been shown to lower blood pressure, a condition most prevalent among men and postmenopausal women. The blood–pressure–lowering effect of walking was acknowledged by Cayce more than half a century ago. In reading 2533–6, Cayce told a patient suffering from hypertension: *"Walk in the open early of mornings. This brings better activity of oxygen and ozone as to keep the balance in the blood flow through lungs, heart, liver, kidneys. These are the sources from which either the pressure or repression causes disturbance."*

Walking is a weight–bearing exercise, in which strain or weight is applied to the bone. Weight–bearing exercise is the most effective method for strengthening bone mass and thus for preventing osteoporosis. Indeed, osteoporosis need not be an unavoidable side effect of menopause and aging. Bone is living tissue that continuously renews and regenerates itself throughout the entire lifespan. Old bone cells break down, and new ones are being built. Mineral salts, including calcium, phosphorus, and magnesium, are continuously being deposited into bone tissue, allowing it to remain hard and unbending. Although the body's bone–building activity slows down somewhat as we get older, it can be increased at any age and maintained at optimal levels through a physically active lifestyle.

Exercise is the only way to stimulate bone–building cells into action. It's also important to provide the body with high–quality raw materials through good nutrition, but it's only through weight–bearing exercise that bone actually gets built. Research has shown that people who are bedridden and unable to stand up lose bone mass very quickly. Bone loss has also been observed in astronauts who returned to earth after spending several days or weeks in space where there was no gravitational pull. Assisted resistance exercises, such as applying pressure to the soles of the feet or the palms of the hands, are a must for anyone who is confined to bed for a considerable length of time. It is only by keeping the pressure on our bones that we can make them strong and resilient. For those who are able to do so, walking is one of the best ways of achieving this.

The Benefits of Exercising Outdoors

Walking also gets us outdoors, into the sunshine and the fresh air, and with today's indoor lifestyles, we often get far too little of both. Cayce suggested that we should *"Supply to the body more action through the general forces of supply to the system outside, close to nature."* (4266–1). Another reading says: *"But long walks morning and evening are well, as to the exercise; and when doing same breathe deep into the lungs."* (272–8) Deeper breathing allows more oxygen to reach deeply into the lungs, replacing stale air that has accumulated during periods of shallow breathing. Because of poor breathing habits, most people use less than a third of their total lung capacity. This means that better breathing could more than double the amount of oxygen that reaches the lungs, the blood, and ultimately the cells of the body. Increased oxygen means increased circulation and better detoxification and nourishment of all body cells.

Outdoor exercise is an excellent way to improve breathing. When the body moves, it demands more oxygen. Breathing should never be forced or choppy, but always gentle and easy, smoothly flowing. Deeper and slower breathing is also the perfect antidote to stress. The fight–and–flight response—the position most of us unconsciously adopt in

response to a perceived stressor—causes muscles to contract and re-
stricts breathing, making it quick and shallow. By consciously altering
the breathing pattern with deeper and slower breaths, it is possible to
relax the entire nervous system in a relatively short time. The deeper
the breath you take, the less often you will need to breathe. The average
person breathes about sixteen times a minute. Those who are skilled in
proper breathing, as are practitioners of Chi Kung, for instance, breathe
only five or six times a minute. The slower and deeper the breathing,
the calmer the person is. He or she is also far less likely to become
breathless or fatigued.

You will notice that your posture plays a significant role in your
ability to breathe well. When you're slouched in a chair or sofa, the rib
cage compresses the lungs, making it difficult to fill them with air. The
more erect you sit or stand, the better your breathing capacity. Deep
breathing, in turn, will strengthen muscles and help them work more
efficiently, thus improving posture. Even the internal organs receive a
workout through proper breathing: the contracting and expanding diaphragm massages the kidneys, liver, stomach, and heart. When the lungs
are expanded on the in-breath, even the intestines and sex organs receive a gentle massage.

Breathing is the most vital of body functions. An improvement in
breathing patterns and breathing capacity brings about an immediate
improvement in all other body functions. Breathing is the very foundation of life, and it enhances the body's ability to regenerate itself. Reading 2072-5 says, *"Breath is the life blood cleansing of the body . . . For, there are the
needs for the combination of the gases as inhaled to act upon the purifying of the
system."*

Exercising outdoors also helps us to spend time in natural sunlight.
Reading 1739-2 suggests: *"Most of the exercise should be outdoors, but not* night.
Day—sunlight—" The "sunshine nutrient," vitamin D, is an essential nutrient for the absorption of calcium and other minerals from the diet.
Vitamin D produced in the skin with the interaction of sunlight is func-
tionally superior to synthetic vitamin D, such as that added to milk and
other fortified foods. Research has shown that residents of northern
latitudes frequently suffer from vitamin D deficiency, especially in the
winter. The elderly are at particularly high risk.

An excellent activity to pursue outdoors is gardening. A study conducted at the University of Arkansas in Fayetteville, U.S., showed that yard work could help to prevent bone–thinning in older women. The researchers found that women who worked in the garden at least once a week had stronger bones than those who were more sedentary.

Outdoor exercise is also important for children and adolescents. Most of the body's bone–building activity takes place in the first twenty years of life. Children's natural urge to run, jump, and play outdoors should therefore be encouraged as much as possible. A study conducted at the University of Tafira in the Canary Islands, Spain, in 2001 identified soccer as an excellent sport for strengthening young men's bones. Researchers found that the long–term participation in soccer helps to boost bone density, thus reducing the risk of fractures and osteoporosis over the long term. Young men who had begun playing soccer before they reached puberty had heavier bones in their legs and spine than those who had been less physically active.

Research studies such as these confirm the energizing, rejuvenating effects of outdoor exercise, as given by Cayce: *" . . . it is the best way to keep yourself young—to stay close to nature, close to those activities in every form of exercise that breathes in the deep ozone and the beauty of nature. For you may breathe it into thine own soul . . . "* (3374–1)

The Head-and-Neck Exercises

Next to walking, the Cayce readings suggest the "head–and–neck" exercises as being of primary importance in maintaining good health. This is a set of gentle bending and rolling exercises of the neck, which help to relieve muscle tension and increase circulation to the head, brain, ears, and eyes. With improved circulation, greater mental clarity, visual acuity, and better hearing ability are often achieved. Cayce reading 3549–1 describes the head–and–neck exercises:

> *Sitting erect, bend the head forward three times, to the back three times, to the right side three times, to the left side three times, and then circle the head each way three times. Don't hurry through with it but take the time to do it.*

This reading also instructs that it is important to keep these exercises on a regular basis if results are to be achieved:

Take this regularly, not taking it sometimes and leaving off sometimes, but each morning and each evening take this exercise regularly for six months and we will see a great deal of difference . . . You will get results.

According to reading 379–16, the benefits of the head–and–neck exercises extend beyond the area of the head and neck to the entire body: " . . . *the head and neck exercises . . . will aid in producing the better balance in the body, or equilibrium, as well as in the circulation to the head and to the heart."* The head–and–neck exercises were sometimes suggested as an aid to become attuned to divine influences in preparation for meditation, or as an aid in relaxing the body before going to sleep at night.

Tinnitus, or a constant sensation of ringing in the ears, is a common complaint of the elderly. The head–and–neck exercises, when done on a regular basis, have proven effective in the relief of this annoying condition. Dr. William A. McGarey has found that these exercises are also helpful in the treatment of arthritis. In *Heal Arthritis: Physically-Mentally-Spiritually*, he writes: "A head–and–neck exercise can be used to bring about greater flexibility in the cervical spine. If used regularly over a long period of time, it will correct the rigidity which sometimes comes about in certain types of arthritis. The hearing and visual acuity of the eyes are both sharpened by using this exercise."

Circling the head three times in both directions is one of the fundamental movements of Tai Chi, an ancient Chinese method of exercising that combines slow, gentle movement with meditation. A number of current studies have identified Tai Chi as an ideal type of exercise that can help older people stay active. Several studies have also found Tai Chi to be effective in relieving arthritis pain. Research published in the September 2001 issue of the *Archives of Physical Medicine and Rehabilitation* showed that Tai Chi Chuan, a special type of Tai Chi, can help to improve circulation.

Better circulation achieved through the head–and–neck exercises helps to properly nourish body cells and keep them young, as Dr. Harold

J. Reilly observes in *The Edgar Cayce Handbook for Health Through Drugless Therapy*, written with Ruth Hagy Brod: *"The head-and-neck exercises . . . if performed faithfully each day, will stimulate the circulation to the entire face, head, and neck; keep the throat and jaw line firm; and prevent the formation of double or multiple chins."*

The head–and–neck exercises, requiring only a few minutes time in the morning and evening, are easily incorporated into a daily routine. The benefits are immense, and the time spent is easily recuperated through the greater physical mobility and mental clarity that help to improve productivity when working on various tasks throughout the day.

Health Stretches

Have you ever watched a baby stretch and yawn? There is an amazing fluidity and suppleness to the stretching movements of very young children, who tend to stretch with utter abandon. They're in no hurry when stretching; they surrender totally to the movements which their bodies naturally and gracefully perform. We should all stretch and yawn before getting out of bed in the morning; if we did, we might be in a better mood when we do get up, and our day may go more smoothly as a result.

Stretching the body and limbs is one of the best ways to stay flexible and keep the muscles tuned. The Cayce readings suggest, *"Stretch the body as a cat would stretch. This is the best exercise to keep [the] body in proportion."* (5271-1) and *"The stretching of the body; not in excess, but as a stretching of the arms, of the limbs—side, circular, forward, up, down. Not just as a setting-up exercise, but stretch the arms high above head—stretch the arms to the front—a swinging motion. Two to three minutes of this each day will make for wonders in the feelings and the activities of the body."* (684-1)

The ancient Indian health system of yoga teaches the importance of stretching the body in the various yoga postures, and in Oriental medicine, stretches of the meridian energy lines are regularly performed as part of a treatment or exercise regimen. In fact, several of the yoga postures prescribe stretches that resemble those recommended in the Cayce readings. Yogis keep their bodies amazingly flexible and youthful through yogic routines.

The exercises that Cayce recommended were often specified to be most beneficial for mornings or evenings. In general, morning exercises were designed to be expansive, with an emphasis on stretching the body upwards and exercising mainly the upper body. *"Mornings—with plenty of air in the room, standing, stretch the body to the full height. Rise on toes and at the same time gently raise the arms, so that there is the exercise of the muscular forces as well as the raising of the structural portion of the body."* (259–10)

The evening exercises were more contractive, with an emphasis on exercising the lower limbs. *"When ready to retire, let the exercise preferably be for the lower limbs; this [is] a movement as of sitting on the floor and walking across or swinging the limbs one in front of the other for three to four movements."* (2454–2)

The morning exercises help to draw the energy upwards in the body in preparation for the day's activities, while the evening exercises help to draw energy and blood flow downwards, away from the head, in preparation for the night's rest and sleep. Reading 288–11 explains: *" . . . the evening exercises for the blood flow away from the head, and of mornings with the upper portion of body. Swinging, circular motion then of lower portion of body in evenings, and the circular motion of hands and upper portion of body of mornings . . . "*

Cayce frequently emphasized the importance of coordinating the breath with the exercise movements. The following reading includes alternative nostril breathing, a technique employed in the yogic tradition to increase pranic (spiritual) energy, and thus health, in the body:

Of morning, and upon arising especially (and don't sleep too late!) - and before dressing, so that the clothing is loose or the fewer the better—standing erect before an open window, breathe deeply; gradually raising hands above the head, and then with the circular motion of the body from the hips bend forward; breathing in (and through the nostrils) as the body rises on the toes—breathing very deep; exhaling suddenly through the mouth; not through the nasal passages. Take these for five to six minutes. Then as these progress, gradually close one of the nostrils (even if it's necessary to use the hand—but if it is closed with the left hand, raise the right hand; and when closing the right nostril with the right hand, then raise the left hand) as the breathing in is accomplished. Rise, and the circular motion of the body from the hips, and bending forward; expelling *as the body reaches the lowest level in the bending towards the floor (expelling through the mouth, suddenly). See?*   1523-2

Today's consumer looking for an exercise program is offered an unprecedented selection of techniques, ancient and modern. There are many different types of yoga, for instance, each emphasizing a different aspect of this ancient Indian health discipline, and each catering to a different personality. Some people like to do vigorous exercises, while others prefer slower, gentler techniques. As we have seen, probably the most important aspect of embarking on an exercise program is that one is able to carry it through and continue doing it persistently. Whether it's walking in the neighborhood park, swimming, cross-country skiing, or dancing, the main thing is to find an activity, or a combination, that you enjoy so that you'll do it because you like it and not because you believe you must.

Putting Stress to Rest with Sleep

During the last part of the twentieth century, stress became a household word. With economic abundance and the multiple choices that result from it, we began having a constant flurry of activities in our lives. To keep ourselves marketable in a competitive work world, we must continuously keep up-to-date on new developments in our field of expertise. Sophisticated technological devices have made communication easier but have also made it easy for us to invade each other's privacy. Private time and family time is frequently interrupted by telephone calls from canvassers and marketing research firms, and our mailboxes are overflowing with unsolicited offers to apply for yet another credit card. Cell phone technology makes sure that we are accessible anywhere, anytime, around the clock. It's almost impossible to book time off. The Internet and e-mail keep us glued to the computer for hours on end, opening up a vast world of information that is wonderfully exciting, but that can also be extremely stressful.

With all this and more going on in our lives, is it any wonder that we feel overwhelmed and unable to cope? When we feel this way, our physical and mental energy starts to crumble and everything around us seems to go wrong. At this point, nothing we can "do" will fix things. The only solution is to get sufficient rest and relaxation. Edgar Cayce put it in very simple terms: *"Unless the body would take time to take care of self, physically and mentally, how* would *one expect to have the correct results from one's activities?"* (349–4) and *"Do not fail to play as well as work. Do not fail to relax mentally and physically."* (257–50)

Research has shown that prolonged mental or physical stress can cause a number of physiological changes, including lowered immune response, high blood pressure, and high cholesterol levels. Stress has also been shown to impair memory by affecting the electrical activity in the hippocampus, the part of the brain that holds on to information. A type of stress, sleep deprivation, also interferes with the forming of new memories and the learning of new skills. Sleep seems to help the brain mold newly acquired information into lasting memories. But the hormones that stress produces in the body seem of themselves to prevent us from getting sufficient sleep, according to a study published in the April 2001 issue of the *Journal of Clinical Endocrinology and Metabolism*. The stimulating effects of corticotrophin–releasing hormone (CRH) were shown to interfere with sleep in middle–aged men worrying about family, work, or finances, perpetuating a seemingly endless cycle of stress, sleep disruptions, and more stress.

If we're caught in such a stress cycle, getting proper sleep is indeed the best remedy. Most people would agree that there is nothing more effective than a good night's sleep to restore body and soul. The trouble for many is that sound, uninterrupted sleep remains an elusive dream. At least one third of the general population suffer from some type of sleep disorder. Even those who don't are often shortchanged when it comes to sleep: With tightly scheduled activities crowding into natural downtime, many individuals sacrifice sleep in order to maximize productivity.

Yet nothing could be more counterproductive. A flood of new research now confirms what our tired bodies and minds have been trying to tell us all along: Sleep is vitally important to our physical, mental, and emotional health. By disregarding our need for sleep, we not only increase our chances of compromising the ability to concentrate, react, and function effectively—we also risk shortening our lives: Those who regularly sleep less than six hours a night don't live as long as those who average seven or eight hours. The sleep–deprived are also more accident–prone and likely to suffer from stress–related illness, including headaches and depression.

The exact nature of sleep is still poorly understood by science, but the benefits of sleep, and the dangers of sleep deprivation, are increasingly coming to light. We know today that sleep is necessary for proper immune function and to help regulate the endocrine system. Sleep–associated processes stimulate the release of important hormones and influence lymphocyte activity. In effect, sleep is a fundamental form of self–regulation for the body.

The phenomenon of sleep has long fascinated philosophers, poets, and mystics. Heine called sleep "the most exquisite of all inventions," and in Shakespeare's Macbeth, sleep is the "balm of hurt minds, great nature's second course, chief nourisher in life's feast." Edgar Cayce referred to sleep as a sixth sense which "acts from the nervous system." (849–20) He explained that there is an "active force within each individual that functions in the manner of a sense when the body–physical is in sleep . . . " (5754–2) As such, sleep directly influences and helps to revitalize and balance the other senses. The central nervous system and its major organ, the brain, are indeed the focus of sleep research, which gained momentum only in the last two decades of the twentieth century.

Sleep Cycles.   By measuring electrical activity in the brain, and by observing eye and body movements, researchers have identified cycles of increased and reduced activity in the brain and body during sleep. One of the most intensely researched stages of sleep is known as REM sleep, which first occurs about an hour or so after we drift off to sleep. REM stands for Rapid Eye Movements, which occur during this phase. Brain activity is high, and the eyes can be seen to move rapidly underneath closed eyelids, while the large muscles in the body are relaxed. This is a deep–sleep phase, during which the sleeper is hard to awaken. Some 80 percent of dreams occur during REM sleep.

REM phases alternate with non–REM (NREM) sleep, when brain activity registers slower wave patterns, which are divided into four distinct phases. The body is most active during the low-frequency delta phase, when sleepers sometimes toss and turn. Those who sleepwalk do so while in delta sleep.

During a typical night, the sleeping individual moves through several cycles of REM sleep, each one of longer duration than the preceding one. The amount of REM sleep is correlated with the amount of mental and emotional stress experienced during the day. When REM sleep is repeatedly interrupted in test subjects, they report feeling nervous and unsure of themselves, which clearly signals that REM sleep, and the dreams that occur during it, are an essential stress–reduction mechanism for the body/mind unit.

Research conducted at the Sleep Research Laboratory at Loughborough University, U.K., has shown that the area of the brain most clearly connected with sleep is the frontal area of the cerebral cortex, which is also responsible for speech, short–term memory, and flexible thinking. As we have noted earlier, short–term memory is one of the main functions to be affected by stress and lack of sleep. As well, a form of schizophrenia is associated with the same part of the brain, and symptoms of sleep–deprivation and schizophrenia are often strikingly similar. The restorative influence of sleep is clearly needed to prevent brain–fog and mental imbalances.

The Chemistry of Sleep.   Folk wisdom holds that babies and children grow during sleep, and modern sleep research has uncovered factors that scientifically substantiate this concept. Researchers at the University of Tennessee have found that a chemical called *growth hormone-releasing hormone* (GHRH) is involved in regulating sleep. Administering the hormone to individuals causes them to sleep longer than they normally would, whereas depriving them of GHRH causes them to sleep less. GHRH stimulates the release of growth hormone, which promotes growth and other metabolic functions, notably protein synthesis. Even after adolescence and throughout adult life, growth hormone continues to be released but in reduced quantities.

Certain neurotransmitters also play an important role in the regulation of sleep. The best known of these is serotonin, which is essential for promoting relaxation and sleep. Neurotransmitters are chemicals used by neurons to signal and stimulate one another. The spaces between nerve cells which facilitate the transmission of signals are called synapses. Researchers believe that one of the reasons why we need to sleep is that sleep exercises these synapses, which lie almost dormant during wakefulness.

Another chemical, the hormone melatonin, which is produced by the pineal gland, has received considerable attention for its role in promoting sleep. Melatonin secretion is regulated by the natural cycle of light and darkness. The use of indoor lights and insufficient exposure to natural sunlight during the day suppress melatonin secretion, resulting in varying degrees of sleep disruption. Our modern lifestyles with their many interferences of the natural sleep/wake cycle appear to be major culprits in preventing us from getting a good night's sleep.

The Circadian Rhythm.   Derived from the Latin "circa diem" (about a day), the circadian rhythm is a twenty-four-hour cycle of physiological and behavioral patterns governed by the body's internal clock, a tiny clump of cells in the hypothalamus known as the suprachiasmatic nucleus (SCN). The SCN is synchronized to light/dark cycles in the environment and other daily cues. In a natural environment, we would sleep when it is dark and be awake and active during the daylight hours. We would sleep longer hours in the winter and much less during the summer months, when nights are shorter. But in order to function as a society, we have imposed artificial, inflexible schedules on ourselves, with the result that our internal clocks are thrown out of sync and can no longer support our natural rhythm.

Window-less office environments with fluorescent lighting fixtures are particularly damaging, but even ordinary household lighting can interfere with the brain's internal clock. A study done at Brigham and Women's Hospital in Boston throws light on why many of us find it so hard to get up in the morning. According to the researchers, exposing people to indoor lighting after sunset shifts the normal time of their peak drive for sleep from about midnight to about 4 or 5 a.m., with the result that they are required to get up much closer to the time when their bodies are making peak demands for sleep.

Folk wisdom and traditional health care methods, notably Ayurveda and Oriental medicine, have long maintained that sleep begun at least an hour before midnight is more refreshing and rejuvenating than sleep extended late into the morning. Modern sleep research is now substantiating this claim. The Cayce readings, too, suggest, "... *don't sleep too late!*" (1523-2) and *"Well that the body rest with the shadows. Early to bed, early to rise."* (4569-1)

The Mystery of Sleep. No sleep study has yet come up with a satisfactory answer to one of life's most fascinating questions: What happens to consciousness during sleep? Does it simply shut down, leaving only a reserve function to produce and process dreams as a figment of the imagination; or does it travel out of the body, eventually returning with memories of its adventures which we then remember as dreams?

Philosophers and mystics have often described sleep as the shadow of death, a reflection of the state when the connection of body and soul is permanently severed. This is illustrated in a quote from *In the Light of Truth: The Grail Message* by Abd-ru-shin: "Even when the gross material body is asleep, its firm union with the soul is loosened, because during sleep the body produces a different radiation, which does not bind so fast as that required for the firm union. But since the union still exists, only a loosening takes place, no separation. This loosening is immediately ended at each awakening." Elaborating on this phenomenon, Dr. Richard Steinpach says in *Why We Live After Death*: "Before achieving deep sleep, some persons have the sensation that they are falling, and they physically twitch. It is the moment when the soul rises out of the previously firm radiation–connection [with the body]." Dr. Steinpach contends that the rapid eye movements observed during deep REM sleep indicate that "the spirit is experiencing a world of higher animation that the sluggish earthly eye is hardly able to follow ... What we describe as dreams are the experiences of spirit in the world beyond."

Edgar Cayce describes sleep as "that period when the soul takes stock of that it has acted upon during [the time between] one rest period to another ... " He says that sleep, as the sixth sense, is the activating force of another, higher "self" which is a "faculty of the soul–body itself ...

When the physical consciousness is at rest, the other self communes with the *soul* of the body . . . " (5754–2) Cayce contends that our thoughts, emotions, attitudes, and actions in the waking state determine our experiences in sleep, when we check in with our higher selves as to whether our activities have been in line with the ideals that we hold at the soul level.

According to Cayce, the moments after an individual first falls asleep are an ideal time for suggestive therapy, particularly in children. During this time, the individual is said to be especially responsive to suggestions being made to the subconscious. Conditions which have been successfully treated with presleep suggestion are wide ranging and include bedwetting, thumb–sucking, and imbalances of the nervous system, such as insomnia itself. In her book *The Miracle of Suggestion*, Cynthia Pike Ouellette recounts how she used presleep suggestion therapy to help her daughter, who was born with multiple disabilities and was not expected to live, yet beat the odds and developed normally despite medical predictions to the contrary.

Getting Better Sleep.   Paradoxically, the quality of our sleep affects our health, but the state of our health also determines how well we sleep. Illness can cause insomnia, and sleep deprivation can cause illness. Not surprisingly, conditions involving severe discomfort, such as osteoarthritis, are frequently associated with insomnia. Indigestion and other digestive problems, notably peptic ulcers, are known to cause insomnia. Hormonal imbalances also account for many hours of lost sleep and may be the main reason why women are 50 percent more likely to suffer from insomnia than men. A 1998 study by the U.S. National Sleep Foundation confirmed that the hormonal changes associated with menstruation, pregnancy, and menopause produce sleep disruptions in the majority of women.

Since digestive system disturbances, particularly liver congestion, have a strong influence on the synthesis and break–down of hormones, it is important to improve digestive function when addressing sleep disorders. Eating the last meal of the day no later than three hours before going to bed helps to prevent digestive discomforts during the night. Avoid fried, greasy foods, and combinations of large amounts of protein and starch at the same meal. These are difficult to digest and likely to cause bloating and gas. It also helps to reduce the consumption of caffeinated beverages—coffee, black tea, and colas; avoid these completely in the late afternoon and evening.

Also high on the list of sleep–promoting activities is physical exercise. Research has shown that those who exercise several times a week fall asleep faster and stay asleep longer than nonexercisers.

Herbal Sleep Aids.   A number of herbal remedies are highly effective in promoting sleep naturally. These are safer than pharmaceutical sleeping pills, which not only create a drug dependency, but also have the counterproductive effect of depressing important REM sleep, thus producing symptoms of REM deprivation, such as confusion and irritability. Herbal relaxants are not habit–forming and have no negative effects on daytime behavior.

One of the most popular herbs for relieving insomnia and anxiety is *valerian root*, whose use dates back to ancient Greece. Throughout Europe, valerian preparations are well–known as a nonaddictive alternative to pharmaceutical sleeping pills. Several research studies have confirmed the ability of valerian root to gently sedate the central nervous system through its action on a group of brain cells known as GABA receptors.

Another favorite herbal sleep aid is lavender, whose essential oil has a relaxing effect on the nervous system through its action, via the olfactory bulb, on the brain's limbic system and the hypothalamus gland. Aromatherapists value lavender for its mood–balancing, antidepressant, and sedative qualities. A 1995 study involving elderly nursing home residents, conducted by the University of Leicester, U.K., concluded that the aroma of lavender worked as well as sleeping pills in helping insomniacs to fall asleep and stay asleep. Test subjects who had been taking pharmaceuticals prior to the study were able to discontinue these when they began using the lavender therapy. Lavender oil placed in an aromatic diffuser or oil burner in the bedroom allows the fragrant molecules to be released into the air. Alternatively, a few drops of the oil can be sprinkled on a pillow or handkerchief placed close to the face.

Other helpful herbs include camomile, linden flower, catnip, and skullcap. Tinctures or teas of these herbs can be taken alone or in combination. A number of effective herbal tea preparations specifically aimed at promoting better sleep are available in natural food stores.

An old folk remedy for insomnia also suggested by Cayce, a glass of hot milk sweetened with unpasteurized honey and taken at bedtime, can be helpful. The easily digested simple sugars in honey promote the conversion of the amino acid tryptophan (found in milk) to the important sleep chemical serotonin.

A bedtime snack of calcium–rich foods, such as almonds, dates, figs, or sesame seeds, also helps to produce a relaxed state in the body. A well–balanced calcium/magnesium supplement is equally effective.

A sleep–friendly environment is also important. Darkness promotes the production of the sleep chemical melatonin. Keeping light out of the bedroom as much as possible is therefore important. The room should be well ventilated and cool, but not cold. Low–frequency fields generated by electrical appliances can interfere with sleep, and it is best to unplug such devices if they are located close to the bed. Some individuals report that their sleeping patterns have improved with the use of a magnetic sleeping pad, which realigns and supports the body's natural magnetic field.

As important as sleep is, more is not necessarily better. Although there are individual variations in the need for sleep, most people function adequately on seven to eight hours a night. This agrees with Cayce's assessment that *"Seven and a half to eight hours should be for most bodies."* (816–1) Researchers at the Department for Sleep Medicine at the University Clinic in Bochum, Germany, say that sleeping excessively can be as damaging as not getting enough sleep. Dr. Michael Bonnet and Dr. Donna Arand of the Kettering Medical Center in Dayton, Ohio, concur. In their opinion, getting more sleep is like gorging on food or drinking to excess. But with today's busy lifestyles and hectic schedules, chances are most of us need not lose valuable sleep worrying about overindulging in this wonderful elixir.

Herbal Remedies: Nature's Own Cures

*Then the motivative element may be within the attributes of nature itself,
whether it be through mechanical applications or medicinal properties or
herbs. Whose herbs are they? Whose force or power is used? They are one!*
Edgar Cayce reading 1620-1

THROUGHOUT HISTORY, HERBAL remedies have been used as medicine. Ancient traditional healing systems such as Traditional Chinese Medicine (TCM) and Ayurveda rely on herbs extensively. Some six thousand different herbs are recorded in the text books of TCM. Few people are aware that even pharmaceutical drugs are often based on herbs. One of the most widely used drugs, *aspirin*, is the chemical version of willow bark, one of nature's great anti-inflammatory herbs. Quinine, used in the treatment of malaria, is a crystalline alkaloid derived from the South American *chinchona* bark. Ipecac, an emetic and expectorant drug that is used to treat accidental poisoning, is prepared from *ipecacuanha*, the root of a South American shrub.

The major difference between herbal remedies and plant-based pharmaceutical preparations is that synthetic drugs are made from the extract of the herb's active ingredient. Herbal tinctures, teas, and powders, on the other hand, are prepared from the whole plant, which ensures that substances that play a synergistic role in the herb's absorption and assimilation are fully preserved. Even though we don't always know what the purpose of those substances is, herbal medicine acknowledges nature's wisdom in combining elements in a certain balance, knowing that nature is not wasteful—these substances would not be there unnecessarily. The isolated "active" ingredients found in pharmaceutical drugs, together with additives and fillers, are more likely to create chemical imbalances and toxicity in the body.

Herbs are plants, and plants have nutritional value. Herbs are sources of vitamins, minerals, and a host of other phytochemicals whose healing potential we are just beginning to understand. In response to a growing interest among drug-weary consumers, we now have more research experiments involving popular herbs such as Echinacea, St. John's Wort, and Green Tea. Sales of medicinal botanicals in North America are growing steadily, amounting to an impressive $4 billion in 1998. Chinese herbs, too, are enjoying increasing popularity in North America. In recognition of this trend, the Hong Kong government, together with the New World China Biosciences Company, began a $1 million research sponsorship project involving two commonly used Chinese herbs, *danshen* and *sanqi*, in the year 2000. This is expected to raise the profile of TCM worldwide, as will other research, such as a study conducted at the University of Illinois at Chicago in 2001, which showed that *ya dan zi (Brucea javanica)*, a popular Chinese herb traditionally used to treat such conditions as fever, dysentery, and warts, was able to ward off the development of cancerous abnormalities in laboratory animals. The university's Natural Inhibitors of Carcinogens Project is further investigating the cancer-preventive properties of *ya dan zi* and other herbs.

Turmeric, a curry spice used extensively for medicinal purposes in Ayurveda, has also been the subject of several recent studies. *Curcumin*, the active substance in turmeric, has been shown to possess anti-inflammatory and anticarcinogenic properties, and has also demonstrated antioxidant activity. Curcumin gives turmeric its distinctive yellow color. Turmeric is a popular spice in traditional East Indian and Asian cuisine, where it is used not only to impart flavor to traditional dishes, but also to preserve their freshness.

Another popular herb and culinary essential in Asian dishes, ginger root, has been the subject of study involving osteoarthritis patients. Research reported in the November issue of the journal *Arthritis and Rheumatism*, showed that patients with osteoarthritis of the knee who took highly concentrated ginger extract noted a significant reduction in knee pain. Herbalists use ginger medicinally to stimulate digestion, improve circulation, and promote detoxification in the body. Ginger also acts to combat nausea, including nausea associated with pregnancy. Research has also shown ginger to be effective in relieving motion sickness. The Cayce readings recommend ginger as an ingredient in several herbal formulations, notably those intended to balance the digestive system.

Several herbs used as spices in ethnic culinary traditions have been shown to promote digestion and possess antioxidant properties, including Vietnamese coriander, rose geranium, winter savory, sweet bay, and oregano. Mexican scientists have also found oregano to slow the growth of bacteria commonly found in food, such as E. coli, S. aureus, and Salmonella.

Interesting studies have also been done with a number of herbs that are traditionally used to relieve hot flashes and other discomfort in menopausal women. Researchers at the Veterans Affairs Medical Center, University of Pittsburgh, Pennsylvania, found that herbs such as black cohosh, blue cohosh, dong quai, red raspberry leaf, licorice root, milk thistle, and ginseng demonstrate estrogenic activity. So, modern science is not only confirming what herbalists and those in the Wise Woman tradition have long known—that these herbs are highly effective—but science is also able to provide an explanation for *why* this effect occurs.

But Mother Nature still guards some of her secrets. Take cranberries, for instance. Several studies have shown cranberries and cranberry juice to be effective in the prevention and treatment of urinary tract infections, which often don't respond to antibiotic treatment, according to research done at the University of Surrey in Guildford, U.K. Cranberries work, but the jury is still out on the specific reason for the popular berry's medicinal effect. Certain chemical compounds in cranberries appear to prevent bacteria, especially E. coli, from adhering to the lining of the bladder and urethra. Some researchers believe that this is due to increased acidity of the urine following cranberry consumption, but others argue that the cranberry's acids are not sufficiently concentrated in urine to be solely responsible for this beneficial effect.

Research conducted at the University of Scranton in Scranton, Pennsylvania, showed that cranberries contain unusually high concentrations of phenols, which are disease–fighting antioxidants. Phenols are also found in other fruits, but out of nineteen commonly consumed fruits, the cranberry had the highest phenol content. Cranberries are also rich in vitamin C, which helps the body to fight off infections.

Clearly, cranberries and their juices are one of Mother Nature's superfoods—a special concentration of nutrients and phytochemicals so well combined that scientists still have not been totally successful in decoding its medicinal secrets.

Green tea, popular in the Japanese tradition, has been shown to have anti–inflammatory effects, due to the action of certain polyphenols that inhibit the expression of a key gene involved in the inflammatory response. Another type of Japanese tea, *oolong*, was found to relieve the symptoms of atopic dermatitis, or eczema. Again, research suggests that polyphenols are responsible for this beneficial effect.

St. John's wort, also known as *hypericum*, has been shown in several studies to be effective in the treatment of depression. An article in the December 11, 1999, issue of the *British Medical Journal* says that St. John's wort was as effective as the antidepressant drug imipramine in reducing depression scores, and it was better tolerated by patients. This was confirmed in another study documented in the September 2, 2000, issue of the same publication. St. John's wort may also help to relieve symptoms of premenstrual syndrome (PMS), including anxiety, nervous tension, and insomnia, according to research reported in the July 2000 issue of the *British Journal of Obstetrics*. In several European countries, St. John's wort is now a licensed medication used to treat depression and anxiety.

My personal favorite is the herb Echinacea, widely used in the healing tradition of North American natives. An alcohol tincture of this herb has helped me and my family numerous times to fight off a cold or flu before it had a chance to take hold. Echinacea is an excellent remedy in the treatment of infectious diseases. It destroys the agents of infection, while simultaneously bolstering the body's defenses by increasing the

white blood cell count. It has a stimulating effect on the lymphatic system and has been shown to increase the ability of lymph to carry waste
tissue away from areas of infection. Echinacea also has anti–inflammatory properties, probably due to its cortisone–like activity. Research has
established Echinacea as a safe herb, even when taken during pregnancy.

Herbs in the Cayce Readings

Numerous Cayce readings contain references to herbs, sometimes
given as ingredients in complex formulations, along with specific instructions for how the herbs are to be gathered, prepared, and administered. In this section, we will take a look at some of the herbs and
herbal formulations most frequently recommended by Edgar Cayce.

**American Saffron, Camomile, Mullein, and Slippery
Elm.**   Teas prepared from these herbs are repeatedly recommended in
the readings, either alone or on an alternate basis, or in combination
with each other, to support and soothe the digestive system and to treat
disorders of the skin, notably psoriasis. Let's look at the specific properties of each of these four herbs:

American saffron (carthamus tinctorius) was the herb most frequently
recommended by Edgar Cayce in the treatment of psoriasis, to balance
the digestive system, promote detoxification, and achieve better coordination between the organs of assimilation and elimination. American
saffron is not true saffron, but is actually the safflower. It costs far less
than true saffron. It is an old home remedy that has traditionally been
used in the treatment of measles and other eruptive skin diseases. Other
indications, according to *Planetary Herbology* by Michael Tierra, C.A., N.D.,
include congested and stagnant blood, poor blood circulation, blood
clots, and lower abdominal pains caused by [menstrual] blood congestion. Tierra lists the active constituents of carthamus tinctorius as including palmitic acid, arachic acid, oleic acid, and linoleic and linolenic
acids—all being essential fatty acids whose deficiencies have been associated with various skin conditions in modern research. In *Healing Psoriasis: The Natural Alternative*, author Pagano says: *"The most beneficial effects*

of [saffron] tea are that of flushing out the liver and kidneys, increasing perspiration, and promoting healing of the intestinal lesions [associated with psoriasis]."

Cayce reading 5545-1 recommends: *"Just before the meals are taken, that of a mild tea of Saffron should be able to coat the whole of the stomach proper. This will aid digestion."*

Camomile, a member of the daisy family, has been valued throughout history as a mild yet highly effective home remedy that relieves nervousness, anxiety, and insomnia. It is soothing to the digestive tract and helps to relieve colic and spasms of the stomach and intestines. It has antiseptic and sedative properties. A weak tea prepared from camomile is safe enough to use with infants. When my son was a baby, I found camomile tea indispensable in helping to relieve his occasional tummy ache. The medicinal effect was almost instant—after taking only two or three teaspoons of camomile tea, his bowels would move immediately and he would settle down.

A camomile bath soothes cranky children and promotes peaceful sleep. As a topical remedy for skin disorders, camomile promotes healing and reduces inflammation. In Europe, where it is a staple in many home medicine chests, camomile is known as a "cure-all." There are two types of camomile—Roman camomile and German camomile. The latter is easier to obtain, has a more agreeable taste, and is a superior source of camomile's pharmacological properties.

Cayce reading 641-7 suggests: *"We would keep to the taking, more often, the Saffron Tea as indicated; and we would change or alternate this at times with Camomile Tea. For these tend to form, in the regular activities of the body, the best in the gastric flows for the intestinal disorder."*

Mullein leaves are an age-old folk remedy for coughs and other chest complaints, and the oil from the Mullein flower is frequently used to alleviate ear problems. In his classic, *Back to Eden*, Jethro Klòss, a contemporary of Edgar Cayce known as the "apostle" of natural healing, says that fomentations from hot mullein tea are a *"splendid remedy [to be] taken internally for dropsy, catarrh, swollen joints"* and that these *"fomentations are good for any kind of swelling or bad sores."* Cayce reading 409-36 says, " . . . *weak Mullein Tea would aid in reducing the tendencies for the accumulation of lymph* *through the abdomen and the limbs."*

According to *The Scientific Validation of Herbal Medicine* by Daniel B. Mowrey, Ph.D., *"Mullein Leaf provides an ounce of mucilaginous protection to mucous surfaces, thereby inhibiting the absorption of allergens through those membranes."* It is feasible that the antiallergenic activity thus achieved, along with mullein's anticongestive action, is the reason why mullein was one of herbs specifically recommended for psoriasis in the Cayce readings.

Slippery Elm Bark, like mullein leaves, possesses mucilaginous properties. It is used as a demulcent and to soothe irritated mucous membranes, including soreness of the throat. Dian Dincin Buchman, author of *Herbal Medicine: The Natural Way to Get Well and Stay Well*, calls slippery elm bark *"an exceptionally healing substance."* Dr. Pagano suggests that *"the slippery elm acts as a protective coating along the inner lining of the upper and lower intestinal tract. This can not only prevent seepage of toxins, but helps the healing process of the thin, porous intestinal walls as well as aid in evacuation."*

In the Cayce readings, slippery elm bark is recommended prepared as a tea, but also as a substance to be chewed: *"The chewing of Slippery Elm would also be well. While it would be necessary that this be done in private, owing to the looks of it, we find that it will be most beneficial to the activity of the glands—the salivary glands as well as those in the pylorus, and in the duodenum also. Swallow the saliva that is indicated in the chewing of same; not the powder, but the bark itself, see?"* (641-7)

More information about American Saffron, Camomile, Mullein, and Slippery Elm and their use in the treatment of skin conditions can be found in Dr. John O.A. Pagano's best-selling book, *Healing Psoriasis: The Natural Alternative*.

Watermelon Seed Tea. This tea is recommended in the readings to help flush out the kidneys: *" . . . the taking of about an ounce of Watermelon Seed Tea in two or three ounces of water—about once a week—will aid in clearing those conditions related to the activities of the lower hepatic circulation—the kidneys; or purify or clear same; and will aid in the assimilating forces from the activities of the pancrean reaction. Prepare same in this manner. Cut or crush about forty to fifty seed, and steep or brew in a pint of water as you would ordinary tea. Then put an* *ounce of the tea in two or three ounces of water and drink. Or, if kept in a cool place, the tea may be taken once or twice a day until the full quantity (the pint) is taken; and then left off for a month or six weeks before being taken again."* (1210–4)

Dr. Pagano says in *Healing Psoriasis: The Natural Alternative*: *"Last, but not least, Watermelon Seed Tea has been known for its effectiveness as a diuretic and has been credited for helping bladder infections for centuries. I suggest this tea to my patients as a substitute for Saffron as an aid in flushing out the urinary system."*

Cayce Herbal Formulations.   The Cayce readings also provided formulations for several herbal tonics, including the following combinations:

• A respiratory inhalant made from tincture of tolu balsam, eucalyptus oil, tincture of benzoin, turpentine oil, and rectified creosote, in a grain alcohol base. This formulation was recommended as a bronchial antiseptic that would help to alleviate lung congestion and stimulate expectorant action.

• A cough remedy and respiratory tonic made from horehound, wild cherry bark, rhubarb, elixir of wild ginger, honey, in a grain alcohol base.

• An intestinal tonic combining wild ginseng, wild ginger, tincture of stilingia, elixir of lactated pepsin, in a grain alcohol base.

• A digestive tonic that was said to be "good for everyone as a spring tonic," and to "assist in clarifying the whole system," containing several cleansing and tonifying herbs, including sarsaparilla root, wild cherry bark, dog fennel, yellow dock root, dogwood bark, and prickly ash bark.

• A revitalizing and energizing tonic that was said to rejuvenate the glandular system and stimulate digestion made from elixir of lactated pepsin, liver extract, black snake root, ginseng, and Atomidine, an aqueous solution of iodine from iodine trichloride. According to the readings, this formulation will help to restore natural color to graying hair.

• An eye tonic consisting of sarsaparilla, yellow dock root, burdock, black haw, prickly ash bark, elder flower, tolu balsam, in a grain alcohol base. The readings suggest that this formulation promotes good digestion and improves circulation throughout the body, improving blood flow and nerve stimulation to the optic tissues. This combination was recommended along with the regular practice of the head and neck exercises (see chapter 4) to improve circulation and consequently strengthen vision.

Herbs and Nutrition for Dental Health

For the care of teeth and gums, Cayce suggested: *"That which is best as a mouth wash for the gums may be found in that of Ipsab. That which is best for the teeth is a combination of salt and soda, which is better than all the concoctions that have been sold in tubes or pastes."* (1131–1) Ipsab is featured in many Cayce readings on dental health. It is a natural solution of prickly ash bark, salt, calcium chloride, iodine trichloride, and peppermint oil. This dental formulation was recommended by Edgar Cayce to prevent and treat gum disease, and as a cleanser for plaque, for purification of the mouth, for tightening up loose teeth, and for improving circulation to the teeth. The readings recommend that Ipsab be massaged into the gums, to neutralize bacteria and fight infection. Ipsab has been used successfully in the treatment of bleeding gums and halitosis.

One of the ingredients in this combination, prickly ash bark, is a Native American medicinal herb that has a long tradition of being used to treat conditions such as rheumatism, ulcers, dysentery, gonorrhea, fevers, and gastrointestinal problems. In agreement with the purpose for which it was prescribed in the Cayce readings, the Native Americans also called the herb "toothache bark." In *The Scientific Validation of Herbal Medicine*, author Mowrey writes about prickly ash bark: *"It is supposed that the plant is a direct nervous system stimulant, operating most likely on the pituitary-hypothalamic pathway, and that most of its medicinal properties are achieved indirectly through stimulation of glandular systems."* Some Cayce readings specify that glandular conditions are involved in teeth and gum problems. Gertrude Cayce, Edgar Cayce's wife, coined the name for the Ipsab formula by lining up the first letters of its main ingredients.

Another product that was often recommended by Cayce for use in combination with Ipsab is *Glyco-Thymoline*, an alkaline mouthwash whose ingredients include eucalyptol, menthol, pine oil, thymol, and sodium bicarbonate. Many Ipsab users find that rinsing the mouth with Glyco-Thymoline after the Ipsab gum massage brings even better results than Ipsab alone and counteracts the acidic effect of the iodine in

Ipsab. Glyco–Thymoline, used as a gargle, is also an excellent remedy for sore throat that brings quick relief. Cayce also suggested that Glyco–Thymoline could be taken internally in minute amounts as a quick alkalizer to remedy overacid conditions in the system and as an intestinal antiseptic.

When discussing the subject of dental health, it is important to point out that saliva plays a considerable role in keeping teeth healthy. Saliva keeps decay–causing acids in check by continuously washing them away from the teeth and neutralizing them before they can cause damage. In addition, minerals such as calcium and phosphorus contained in saliva help to repair minor damage to tooth enamel on a continuous basis. Many prescription drugs, including *clonidine*, a medicine used to treat high blood pressure in adults and attention deficit hyperactivity disorder (ADHD) in children, restrict saliva flow, causing dry mouth in those who take them. Less saliva in the mouth means a reduced repair capacity for minor tooth enamel damage, and increased chances for cavities.

The good news is that saliva–inhibiting medication is not the only way to treat high blood pressure and ADHD. Natural treatments, without side effects, are available. One of the most effective therapies in each case is a natural whole foods diet free of refined sugars, which will also help to build healthy teeth and gums.

Prevention of tooth decay and gum problems must begin in childhood, ideally before a baby is born. A baby's teeth begin to form in utero, although they don't fully develop until they start pushing through the gums, sometime between seven and twelve months of age. The mother's nutrition during the months of tooth formation can greatly influence the health of her baby's teeth.

Although the primary (baby) teeth are in some sense "temporary," because they are eventually replaced by the permanent teeth, their role in determining the health of the future permanent teeth should not be underestimated. Primary teeth encourage the normal development of jaw bones and muscles. They also ensure that there is space for the permanent teeth to grow into, and they help guide them into position. The healthier a child's baby teeth are, the stronger his or her permanent teeth will be. Many parents underestimate the importance of keeping the primary teeth healthy, but research has shown that children with cavities in primary teeth are at greater risk of future tooth decay involving their permanent teeth.

Most children start losing their primary teeth between the ages of six and eight, but some baby teeth stay in the mouth until age twelve. The permanent teeth help to push the primary teeth out and then take their place. Tooth formation is thus an ongoing process from the time before birth until well into the teenage years. A nutritious diet, along with high-quality supplements, during these years sets the stage not only for dental health in childhood, but throughout adulthood as well.

The most important nutrient for teeth is calcium, found in green leafy vegetables, egg yolks, dried beans, almonds, sesame seeds, seaweeds, and some root vegetables, especially carrots grown in organic, mineral-rich soil. Dairy foods are also a good source of calcium, but they can be difficult to digest because of mandatory pasteurization, which destroys enzymes. Fermented dairy products, such as yogurt, buttermilk, and kefir, are easier to digest and are especially recommended because their lactic acid content promotes calcium uptake in the small intestine. Always buy full-fat dairy products, especially for children. Low-fat dairy products are not whole foods. The fat in cream and whole milk is an important catalyst which helps the body to assimilate calcium.

The calcium supplement most often recommended in the Cayce readings, notably for pregnant women, is Calcios, which in Cayce's time was made from pulverized chicken bones. Calcios is still available today, but is now produced from cattle bone and marrow. Chewing the soft ends of chicken bones to increase dietary calcium intake was also advised in the readings. For babies and children, Cayce also recommended small amounts of limewater, an aqueous preparation of calcium hydroxide.

Magnesium and vitamin D are required for calcium to be properly assimilated in the body. Magnesium is found in chlorophyll-rich green vegetables, whole grains, legumes, honey, molasses, dates, and nuts, especially almonds, cashews, and brazil nuts. Fish and sea kelp are also good sources. Vitamin D is produced in the body through the interaction of sunlight with certain chemicals in the skin's fatty tissue. Food sources of vitamin D are fish and fish liver oils, and eggs and dairy products.

According to a poll conducted in 2001 by the American Academy of Periodontology, most periodontists believe that a healthy diet, as well as certain supplements, improve the health of teeth and gums. Keeping teeth healthy throughout one's lifetime has a definite impact on the quality of life, especially in the golden years, according to a Japanese survey conducted in 2002. Those over sixty–five who felt that their chewing ability was good also felt that they were in good health, enjoyed a high quality of life, and were able to follow conversation easily. Those who had problems chewing because of dental problems rated their quality of life considerably lower.

The Fluoride Question.   Is fluoride important for dental care? If we believe the TV commercials, dental health in children and adults depends on added fluoride in toothpaste. In addition, many dentists recommend that children take fluoride supplements internally to help build stronger teeth. But holistically oriented dentists disagree. While there is some evidence that the external application of fluoride to tooth enamel provides protection against cavities, the benefits of taking it internally are questionable.

Some researchers warn that fluoridated water increases the incidence of degenerative conditions such as cartilage calcification and bone demineralization. Mottling of teeth, indicated when white or brownish spots appear on tooth enamel, often develops with excessive fluoride consumption. Increasingly, this condition is observed in children. In Canada, the Canadian Dental Association has revised its guidelines and now advises against fluoride supplements in young children, admitting that the evidence supporting the effectiveness of fluoride supplements is weak. But in many North American municipalities, we continue to put fluoride in our drinking water, a practice which is banned in most European countries because of its dangers to human health and the environment.

Many consumers who are concerned about ingesting fluoride in drinking water opt for bottled spring water as one of the few fluoride–free alternatives. A home filtration system based on activated carbon filters does not remove fluoride, but reverse osmosis filtration does. The distillation process removes fluoride, but also removes all healthful minerals from the water (*see the section on Hydrotherapy in chapter 3 for additional information on water treatment options*).

Even after children's teeth are fully developed, and throughout adulthood, good nutrition and a healthy lifestyle play an important role in keeping them strong and healthy. A diet consisting of natural whole foods helps to ensure a healthy mouth flora, which protects against the acids that cause tooth decay. Foods rich in vitamin C help to protect gums against periodontal disease such as gingivitis.

Refined sugars and candies of all kinds should be avoided. Not only do they increase acids locally in the mouth, but they also undermine tooth health by interfering with the assimilation of minerals in the body. Raw or unpasteurized honey, often recommended by Cayce, may be the safest sweetener when it comes to tooth health: New research shows that honey prevents the growth of dental plaque bacteria believed to be responsible for dental caries.

A great deal of research is being done to develop new types of dental fillings that will be able to prevent further tooth decay, and possibly even reverse decay. But in the meantime, superior nutrition and a natural dental care program can help ensure good dental health from infancy to golden age.

Herbal First Aid

Cuts, bruises, fevers, toothaches, abdominal cramps—are you prepared to deal with a minor health emergency at home?

Many herbs found in nature are excellent first-aid remedies that empower us to promptly and effectively respond to minor emergencies and to reduce our dependency on an already overburdened health care system. Herbal first-aid remedies do not prevent us from seeking medical help where appropriate, but they can help to contain a situation that might otherwise develop into a serious crisis. In many cases, they can even resolve the problem without medical intervention.

Our grandparents and great-grandparents were much more self-reliant than we are today in dealing with various ailments. Their simple home remedies were often as close as the kitchen cupboard or herb garden. Modern naturopathy, herbology, and homeopathy derive many of their most effective medicines from such traditional remedies. The following is a list of conditions, along with the appropriate remedies to keep on hand in a well-stocked natural home medicine chest:

Asthma Attack.   The antispasmodic properties of *cranberries* can ease breathing. Keep a batch of cooked, mashed cranberries in the fridge; when needed, stir a teaspoon of the paste into a cup of warm water and drink slowly. *Hot compresses* applied to the back and chest help to relax the bronchi. *Steam inhalations* are also effective in relieving asthma attacks. Add a few drops of eucalyptus, pine needle oil, or wintergreen to a bowl of hot water and inhale. Alternatively, rub the oils on the chest.

For help with bronchial conditions, the Cayce readings frequently recommend inhaling the fumes of apple brandy from a charred oak keg. These fumes help to clear the lungs of congestion while stimulating the circulation of the entire respiratory systems. Cayce reading 5053-1 says: *"This will act not only as an antiseptic, but will so change the lung tissue as to bring about healing of the lung tissues, and will also increase the abilities of assimilation, and we will have improvement."* Dr. John Pagano says that he has witnessed outstanding results with patients who have used the charred oak keg therapy for respiratory conditions.

A pleasant-tasting yet highly effective herbal formulation often suggested in the readings as a cough syrup and respiratory tonic is a mixture of wild cherry bark syrup, syrup of horehound, syrup of rhubarb, and elixir of wild ginger.

Bites and Stings.   *Tea tree oil* or *aloe vera gel* are effective in reducing pain and swelling from mosquito bites. A poultice made with *calendula* or a slice of *raw onion* relieves the pain of a bee sting. Apply a poultice made with *papaya enzyme* to a wasp or hornet sting. Apply essential oil of *lavender* in small amounts directly to the site of the sting. Dr. Pagano has found a mixture of sodium bicarbonate and apple cider vinegar to be an effective remedy in case of insect bites.

Bleeding.   A small amount of *cayenne pepper*, sprinkled on a cut or wound, will stop bleeding quickly. For internal bleeding, a pinch of cayenne taken in a large glass of water, has been shown to be effective.

It is important, however, to obtain medical help as soon as possible for any kind of internal bleeding. Diluted *lemon juice* also helps to stop bleeding. It will sting on application, but is extremely effective. For nosebleeds, soak a cotton ball with fresh lemon juice and insert into the bleeding nostril.

Bruises.   The most popular remedy for any type of bruising is *arnica* cream. It can be applied directly to the affected area, being careful not to massage it too firmly. If it is a particularly bad bruise, it helps to take a supplement of *niacin* (vitamin B3), which increases circulation by dilating the capillaries, and to perform a gentle massage with arnica over the area, directing the flow toward the heart. Homeopathic dilutions of arnica are helpful when taken internally, as well. Depending on the severity, several doses may need to be taken; follow the instructions on the package.

Cold compresses with *apple cider vinegar* or solutions of *witch hazel, comfrey,* or *calendula,* are effective in reducing swelling and soreness.

Note: In the event of a severe bruise suffered from a bad fall or blow, internal hemorrhages may be present which may require medical attention.

Burns.   An excellent burn remedy is *aloe vera* gel, applied directly to the wound. The fresh gel from an aloe plant leaf is best, but bottled gels available in health food stores can be equally effective. Aloe vera is an incredibly versatile first-aid remedy that is effective for many conditions ranging from insect bites and canker sores to herpes and warts. Sunburned skin, too, responds well to treatment with aloe vera.

Dian Dincin Buchman's Herbal Medicine suggests poultices of peeled and cut raw (white) potatoes for burns or scalds.

Essential oil of *lavender* shows remarkable ability to heal burns quickly. In 1928, the French chemist Gattefossé accidentally discovered that lavender was able to rapidly heal a severe burn on his hand and prevent scarring. In *The Fragrant Pharmacy,* author Valerie Ann Worwood recommends soaking a sterile gauze or clean cotton cloth in ice-cold water, then adding one drop of lavender, camomile, or yarrow, or a mixture of these oils, for each square inch of skin affected, and applying it to the area.

Poultices of *raw, unpasteurized honey* have also been successfully used in the treatment of burns.

Drink plenty of water to avoid dehydration.

Colds and Flu.   *Echinacea* tincture is one of the most effective remedies for colds and influenza. At the onset of symptoms, take thirty drops in a small amount of water every half hour or so until symptoms subside. Then reduce the dosage. *Zinc* lozenges soothe a sore throat and speed recovery. Research has shown that taking about ten zinc lozenges (containing 23 mg of zinc) per day reduced the length of recovery from an average eleven to four days. *Cayenne, Ginger,* and *Garlic* are excellent cold-fighters. Add them fresh to foods, or take them in capsule form or as a tea.

A hot drink of pure water or herbal tea, taken with fresh lemon juice and a teaspoonful of *raw honey* is another time-honored cold and flu remedy. Steam inhalations with oils of *eucalyptus* and *pine needle* help to relieve nasal and bronchial congestion associated with colds. Or sprinkle a few drops of the oils in an aromatic diffuser or burner. *Goldenseal* in tincture or capsule form works well for sinus congestion and infection.

Hot baths with the above oils, or *Epsom salts,* are also recommended. Relieve a sore throat by gargling with salt water or *Glyco-Thymoline* (see section on Herbs and Nutrition for Dental Health).

Constipation and Indigestion.   A teaspoonful of *psyllium hulls,* taken in a large glass of water two to three times daily, works wonders in relieving a sluggish intestinal system. Be sure to follow with another large glass of water immediately afterwards, and drink at least eight to ten glasses of water throughout the day.

A tincture of *bitter herbs,* taken in water or herbal tea, relieves bloating, indigestion, and other intestinal complaints. Formulations of bitter herbs are available in natural food stores or specialty pharmacies.

Warm *castor oil* packs, applied over the abdominal area, relieve many types of intestinal stress and rejuvenate the entire digestive system. Soak a folded cloth of wool or cotton flannel in the warmed oil, apply over the abdomen, then cover with a sheet of plastic. Put a towel over the area, then apply an electric heating pad. Leave on for an hour. Afterwards, wash the area with warm water and baking soda, to remove any stickiness (*see chapter 4 for more in-depth information on castor oil packs*).

Dried fruit, especially *prunes* and *figs*, have a laxative action. Raw or cooked *apples*, which provide high–quality fiber in the form of pectin, are also helpful.

Teas of *camomile, peppermint, fennel*, or *ginger* are helpful for relieving many digestive complaints.

Note: If an intestinal obstruction is suspected, seek medical help immediately.

Cramps and Muscle Spasms.   Supplements of *calcium* and *magnesium* may bring relief. Apply *eucalyptus oil* or *arnica* cream, or compresses of *apple cider vinegar*. If the cramp is in the foot or leg, it helps to take a firm step on a cold surface with the affected (barefoot) limb.

For severe cramps in the stomach or abdomen, acupuncturists recommend putting *hot water* continuously on the point on the foot located between the second and third toe (acupuncture point ST–44) until the pain subsides. This is also recommended for sleeplessness and headaches.

Cuts. (See also **"Bleeding"**)   *The Natural Family Doctor* by Dr. Andrew Stanway suggests that bleeding from cuts can be arrested by applying pressure for a few minutes. If the edges of the cut gape open, draw them together firmly with finger and thumb and apply strips of surgical tape. Cover the wound with a dressing and bandage. A minor wound is best left uncovered.

Aloe vera gel, oil of lavender, and *witch hazel* all have antiseptic properties and are recommended in the treatment of cuts.

Diarrhea.   Alternately apply *hot* and *cold compresses*, or warm *castor oil packs* (see "Constipation") over the abdominal area. Avoid dehydration by taking plenty of *liquids*. Drink teas of *peppermint* or *linden flower*. Eat cooked *brown rice* or *barley*, or drink the strained cooking water. Barley water is a time–honored home remedy for controlling diarrhea in infants. Lactic–acid fermented milk products, such as *yogurt* or *kefir*, help to recolonize the friendly bacteria in the intestinal tract.

Note: Seek medical help for prolonged, severe diarrhea, especially in small children and the elderly.

Earaches.   A drop or two of *warm castor oil, olive oil,* or *mullein oil* in the affected ear is an effective remedy in many cases. Put a peeled *garlic* clove wrapped in gauze or cheesecloth in the outer ear canal and leave it there for a few hours or overnight. Hot poultices of steeped and strained *camomile* flowers are also effective in alleviating earaches.

The Cayce readings suggest that earaches are often caused by congestion and inadequate lymphatic circulation in the areas of the head and neck. Any treatment that helps to improve the circulation of blood and lymph in these areas—massage, hot compresses, the head–and–neck exercises (*see chapter 4*)—will also be effective in relieving the earache.

Note: Persistent earaches, especially in young children, may be due to infection and require medical attention.

Fevers and Infections.   Fevers are part of the body's self–healing mechanism and should not be suppressed unless dangerously high. Stay well hydrated by drinking plenty of *liquids*, such as water with lemon juice, herbal teas, light miso soups, or vegetable broths. Drinking *aloe vera juice* is also helpful. Cool off the body by sponging with *cold water*, or applying cold water wraps. In cases of very high fevers, a cool enema helps to reduce internal body heat. *Echinacea, goldenseal,* and *propolis* are effective remedies with a natural antibiotic action.

Note: Persistent high fevers may require medical attention.

Headaches and Migraines.   Many migraine sufferers experience relief by lying down in a darkened room. The application of heat or cold, by means of a *hot water bottle* or an *ice pack*, to the back of the neck also helps. For stress–related headaches or any kind of pain, shiatsu therapists recommend applying *pressure* to the point on the hand deep in the area between the thumb and forefinger (acupuncture Point LI–4), for as long as necessary. For severe headaches which are localized on one side of the head, Ayurvedic practitioners recommend putting a few drops of *salt water* in the nostril on the opposite side to where the pain is felt (e.g., right–side pain/left nostril). Massaging a drop of essential oil of *lavender* or *peppermint* in the area around the temples and back of the neck can bring relief. For nervous headaches, blend lavender with camomile. The Cayce readings recommend a mixture of equal parts of spirit of camphor, tincture of lobelia, and alcohol, as an effective headache rub.

Note: Many headaches are due to digestive disturbances, spinal misalignments, and muscle tension. For the long–term relief of chronic headaches, these conditions need to be corrected. Nutritional detoxification, castor oil packs, and colonic irrigation (*see chapter 3*) are some of the methods suggested in the Cayce readings for relief.

Pain. (See also **Headaches and Migraines**) *White willow bark*, from which salicin, the forerunner of aspirin, is derived, is an effective analgesic for many aches and pains, including headache, rheumatic, and neuralgic pains. This herb can be taken internally in capsule form. Arthritic and rheumatic pains can also be alleviated with *cayenne* poultices.

For back pain and sore muscles, *Tiger Balm*, a prepared herbal ointment, is highly effective. Tiger Balm increases circulation to the affected area and promotes healing by relaxing the muscles. Massage oils containing witch hazel, tincture of benzoin, and sassafras oil were often commended in the Cayce readings to be used as a liniment for tired or aching muscles.

Sprains. For a sprained joint or strained muscle, elevate the affected area, and apply ice and pressure to keep inflammation down and minimize pain. *Arnica* rubs are also recommended. Drink *burdock* tea, and/or apply a poultice of burdock leaves or chopped *raw onion*. Compresses of *apple cider vinegar* are also helpful. Soak the affected area in water to which *ginger* (chopped fresh or ginger tea) has been added.

Toothache. Be sure to dislodge any trapped food particles in a cavity or gum pocket. Rinse well with salt water. Chew on a few *cloves*, or apply *oil of cloves, peppermint*, or *camomile*, to the affected area on the gums. A few grains of *cayenne* powder placed on the gums and tooth also provide relief. Rub a few drops of *Ipsab* (see the section *Herbs and Nutrition for*

Dental Health in this chapter) on the affected area.

For pain from inflammation, try a homeopathic remedy of *camomila* (30C). For nerve pain, try *hypericum* (30C).

Vomiting. In *Natural Family Doctor*, Dr. Andrew Stanway recommends to lie flat and not to eat or drink anything for a couple of hours. Then try small amounts of iced water, or the cool, strained *water from boiled rice* to settle the stomach. As soon as possible, drink plenty of liquids to replace lost body fluids. Drink *peppermint* or *ginger* tea. Homeopathic remedies include *ipecac* and *nux vomica*.

Note: Homeopathic remedies are a very effective first-aid medicine. As remedies are quite specific, check with a qualified homeopathic practitioner. Some excellent homeopathic first-aid kits are also available in health food stores.

Herbal remedies from Mother Nature's pharmacy offer great hope of healing in a world that has become poisoned by the excessive and often inappropriate use of synthetic pharmaceutical drugs. However, even natural remedies can have a powerful effect, and it is always wise to use caution in the treatment of any condition. Biochemical individuality is always to be considered, even when a natural herbal therapy is used. For the treatment of any illness with herbs, it is best to consult a qualified herbalist or naturopathic physician. Cayce reading 2072-6 points out what we would all do well to remember—each person may react differently to herbal preparations: " . . . *remember, each body is a law unto itself respecting such preparations or herbs or minerals from which drugs are made. And these may only be given—that is, as to their beneficial or harmful reactions—in reference to this body.*" (2072-6)

Note: Many of the items mentioned in this chapter are available through Baar Products, the official worldwide supplier of Edgar Cayce health care products. They may be reached through their Web site, www.baar.com, or by calling 610-873-4591 or 1-800-269-2502.

6

Energy Medicine: Subtle Healing Vibrations

Know that all strength, all healing of every nature is the changing of the vibrations from within—the attuning of the divine within the living tissue of a body to Creative Energies.   Edgar Cayce reading 1967-1

WHETHER WE TAKE a medicinal substance in the expectation that it will bring healing or we simply pray that healing be provided by God—in either case, the substance or the prayer serves as an instrument for attunement. Both the medicine and the prayer introduce a healing energy that initiates a change in the body–mind of the patient. The degree to which healing actually takes place depends as much on our willingness to accept healing as it does on the therapy that is used. Whether we begin in the physical dimension by applying medicinal substances or we turn to the spiritual dimension by using prayer—healing is experienced only through a shift in consciousness in the body–mind.

The Cayce readings say, *"Each entity is a part of the universal whole."* (2823-1) We live in a holographic universe, in which a change in a small part of the whole affects the larger, entire whole. Our physical bodies are a part of this holographic universe, and this explains why a physical remedy will affect simultaneously the physical, the mental, the emotional,

116

and the spiritual body. Similarly, a slight shift in the spiritual dimension will manifest in a corresponding shift in the physical, mental, and emotional bodies. The dimension from which healing can most easily be initiated and precipitated depends on the total consciousness of the person. Those who are strongly focused on the physical dimension may not be able to get well without some kind of physical remedy—a medicine they can take or a physical treatment they can undergo. Others whose attention is focused primarily on spiritual influences will feel more comfortable with, and better respond to, a prayer ritual or an energy treatment. Neither is in itself better or worse, and each will affect the whole person. The truly holistic quality of the Cayce readings is evident in the fact that they consistently address all aspects of being—physical, mental, emotional, and spiritual.

But the overall message of the readings strongly emphasizes the concept that we are spiritual beings who have come to temporarily reside in a physical body, which is shaped and molded through the influence of the spiritual energies that we contribute from our spiritual essence. This spiritual energy is transmitted and fed to the physical body in the form of thoughts via the creative building force that is the mind. The readings say: " . . . *the spirit is life; the mind is the builder; the physical is the result.*" (349-4) So everything starts on the mental level, whether it's illness or health. However, the readings also acknowledge that it is possible for physical influences to weaken the mental energies and that therefore some therapeutic action must be taken on the physical level. Ultimately, however, the healing will come from the spiritual dimension, from "within":

> *There may be* applied *mechanical forces as will* aid, *yet the* healing—*the* correction—*the* changes *wrought*—must *be within self and self's own mental forces, and self's own reaction* to *the conditions; for, as in any healing, the* incentive *must be present.*   412-1

The incentive that is emphasized in this reading is sometimes referred to as the desire to not only get well, but also to be "good for something," to have a purpose larger than oneself for becoming healed and whole. Reading 572-5 says: " . . . *begin to plan as to what the body will* do

when and as the improvements come . . . Not only be good; be good for something!
Hold to that which is of Truth!"

The various healing techniques that use energy medicine in its di-
verse disciplines all work on several levels—mental, emotional, spiritual, and physical—to bring about a vibratory change that realigns a
person's energies to resonate with health rather than illness. They can
accomplish their task all the better if the patient has an incentive for
getting better and a spiritual ideal, as often suggested in the readings.

Vibrational healing can be accomplished through the senses, such as
smell, sight, sound, and touch; through magnetic force; through the
chakras, which are the body's energy vortices; or through the energies
of prayer and meditation. In the pages that follow, we will look at several different techniques of energy healing, and at some of the Cayce
readings that also recommended them. Prayer and meditation are discussed separately in chapter 7.

Aromatherapy's Fragrant Healing Energies

One of the ways in which we can introduce specific healing energies
into our environment is with aromatherapy, which employs aromatic
fragrances to subtly alter body chemistry and mood. For instance, if
you're feeling stressed out, exhausted, and lethargic, you can give your
energy level a boost by surrounding yourself with the fragrant oils of
rosemary, peppermint, or jasmine. Or, if you are nervous, unable to
relax, and plagued by insomnia, try the soothing scents of lavender,
sweet marjoram, or camomile, and feel your tension melt away. Could
healing be that simple? As close as your nose?

The use of aromatic plant essences to balance physical, emotional,
and spiritual energies, enjoys growing popularity today. The benefits of
aromatherapy are valued in therapeutic massage and professional skin
care. And as scientific research substantiates the effectiveness of essential oils in alleviating a number of common ailments, aromatherapy
holds great promise for medical applications, especially in the developing field of psychoneuroimmunology.

Edgar Cayce often recommended essential oils in massage, baths, and
inhalations, for conditions ranging from nervous disorders and bron-

chial catarrh to tuberculosis. The readings also provided fascinating in-
sights into the multidimensional effects of fragrance, including its potential for promoting spiritual attunement and the manifestation of
latent talents and inclinations resonating from a previous life.

In reading 346–1, Cayce suggested that the burning of incense may
help a textile research consultant tap into mental abilities developed
during a past life in Egypt at the time of Ra Ta: *"Hence those things oriental,
those things that deal with subtle odors, subtle activities upon those senses of individuals, play their part in the experience of the entity; and—not sandalwood, but—
cedar surrounding the entity will bring a satisfaction; and in the burning of same, in
the odors of same, may the entity harken back to much of the developed mental
abilities of the entity, for the series of activities that the entity may seek to find in its
relationships to individuals, to itself, to solving problems; and always burn* three,
when such is done."

Aromatic plant essences have been in use for thousands of years,
both for religious and medicinal purposes. In ancient Egypt, perfumes
were believed to be emanations from deities, serving both to announce
the imminent manifestation of a god or goddess, and to enable worshippers to enter into the realms of the nether-world, the dwelling place
of the gods. The mystical aspect attached to fragrances had considerable
significance in ancient Egypt. Some metaphysically oriented Egyptolo-
gists subscribe to the theory that the anatomical structure of the nasal
cavity is reflected in the architecture of the Temple of Luxor, whose
secret sanctuary chambers are presumed to represent the olfactory, pineal, and pituitary glands in the human head.

In many Eastern religions, as well as in the Catholic Church, fragrance in the form of incense continues to be widely used in a ritualistic
or ceremonial manner to facilitate attunement to Spirit.

The Physiology of Scent.   As their name implies, essential oils
carry the essence of a plant's specific energy pattern. The oils are stored
in the blossoms, leaves, stems, or roots, where their concentration var-
ies depending upon the time of day and year. Accordingly, herbalists
carefully choose the season, as well as the hour, for harvesting the plants.
The soil and the climate in which a plant is grown also significantly
influence the composition of the plant's biochemical constituents.

The unique chemical make-up of each plant oil is characterized by its special fragrance, which we perceive when airborne odor molecules enter the nasal passages and stimulate the tiny olfactory hairs (cilia) on the nasal epithelium. The sense of smell is unique among the senses because it allows us to instantly reconstruct memories involving all other senses, including sight, sound, and touch. As if it held the key to a hologram, a familiar scent virtually brings memories to life.

This reaction occurs because signals from the olfactory cilia are transmitted to the brain's limbic cortex, the oldest part of the brain in human evolution, which acts as a storehouse for memories of past experiences involving pleasure, pain, and other feelings. In addition, the limbic system controls most involuntary aspects of behavior, primarily through the hypothalamus gland, which also regulates the secretion of the pituitary hormones. This explains why fragrance is effective in altering moods and emotional states, as well as in initiating chemical reactions within the body. Research conducted at the University of Nottingham, U.K., showed that certain odors could trigger pathological symptoms in veterans of the 1991 Gulf War. Smells of diesel or tar, for instance, could bring on poor concentration, migraine-type headaches, or muscle fatigue. A 2001 study at the University of Calgary in Alberta, Canada, showed that emotionally charged memories were more likely to be evoked through odor than memories associated with a more neutral state of mind. Fragrance-triggered memories can be painful as well as pleasant.

Mystical Lavender.   Edgar Cayce acknowledged the considerable influence of environmental odors, when, at the beginning of reading 1551-1, he spontaneously commented: *"You know, it would be very well for the body to change the odors about the room from almond to lavender, and it would be much better."*

The light, balsamic scent of lavender has long been popular as a home fragrance and as a closet and bathroom freshener. But even more remarkable is lavender's medicinal value. Known in France and throughout other parts of Europe as an indispensable home remedy for bruises, bites, and minor aches and pains, oil of lavender is also a popular ingredient in many therapeutic essential oil formulations. In fact, the term *aromatherapy* owes its existence to lavender. It was coined in 1928 by the French chemist *Gattefossé*, after he accidentally discovered that oil of lavender promoted rapid healing of a severe burn on his hand, and also prevented scarring. Aromatherapists today value lavender for its antiseptic and antibiotic properties, and for its mood–balancing, antidepressant, and sedative qualities.

The Cayce readings provide a mystical explanation for the transformational effects of lavender in reading 274–10, describing lavender as *"that upon which the angels of light and mercy would bear the souls of men to a place of mercy and peace, in which there might be experienced more the glory of the Father."*

Aromatherapy in Massage.   Cayce also recommended lavender as an ingredient in massage oil formulations, to promote circulation and lymphatic drainage. Therapeutic massage is a highly effective method for applying essential oils. When massaged into the skin, the molecules of plant essences contained in the massage oils are absorbed through the pores and transported through the blood stream via the tiny capillaries located in the tufts beneath the epidermis. The kneading and stroking motions applied during the massage simultaneously increase blood flow to the tissues, thus ensuring optimal absorption of the aromatic essences.

Because plant oils are highly concentrated, they must be diluted and combined with a carrier oil before they come in contact with the skin. A high–quality vegetable oil, such as grape–seed, almond, or jojoba, is usually preferred. Only a few drops of the essence are required to yield an effective product.

Baths and Inhalations.   Essential oil can also be added to bath water, undiluted or combined with vegetable oil (ten drops of essence to a teaspoon of carrier oil). The warmth of the water allows the pores to open, facilitating absorption of the plant essences by the skin. Simultaneously, the medicinally effective aromatic vapors released with the steam are inhaled into the lungs. Stimulant oils such as rosemary, peppermint, jasmine, and clary sage, are usually preferred for an invigorating morning bath, while the calming effects of sweet marjoram, camomile, lavender, and valerian make for a relaxing soak at bedtime.

For those suffering from arthritis or bronchial disturbances, Edgar Cayce often suggested the addition of pine needle oil to the bath. Pine needle oil was also recommended for inhalations, usually in combination with eucalyptus oil. Reading 973–1 says: *"Keep the fumes in the room, to be inhaled, from boiling equal parts of Oil of Eucalyptus and Oil of Pine Needles; that is, boil these (in water) in the room, so that the fumes may be inhaled. These will be strengthening."* Eucalyptus is a common ingredient in natural remedies formulated to combat the common cold and nasal or bronchial congestion. It is also used clinically in France, where research has shown that eucalyptus kills up to 70 percent of staphylococcal bacteria.

The skin, too, benefits from facial steam baths. Lemon, cypress, and mint have astringent qualities and help to cleanse and tighten the pores of oily skin, while lavender, clary sage, and neroli will smooth out wrinkles in mature skin and promote cell regeneration. Combined with a good base oil like almond, avocado, or apricot kernel, these essences can also be made into a nourishing facial oil, which is great for a relaxing facial massage at home, or serves as an effective substitute for commercial night creams.

A few drops of essential oil added to a mild shampoo or conditioning rinse can help improve hair texture and highlight the natural hair color. For light hair, add camomile, lemon, or golden rod; for dark hair, use rosemary, rosewood, or sandalwood; for dandruff problems, try thyme, cedarwood, or tea tree oil.

A Fragrant Environment.   An easy and pleasant way to enjoy the benefits of aromatherapy is to vaporize a few drops of essential oil in an aromatic diffuser or oil burner. Citrus oils, such as citronella or lemongrass, quickly remove stale cigarette smoke or cooking odors, and are also effective as insect repellents. Peppermint, lemon, grapefruit, or sage promote mental alertness by "energizing" the air, while the soothing scents of lavender and camomile promote relaxation and a peaceful atmosphere at the end of a busy day. In research experiments, camomile has been demonstrated to have a sedative effect on the subjects, while also elevating their mood and decreasing their emotional responsiveness to suggested negative imagery, indicating a strengthened "emotional immune system."

When we view current–day research pertaining to essential oils from the perspective of the Cayce readings on the effects of fragrance, we catch a glimpse of the tremendous healing potential of aromatherapy. Through harmonizing body energies, stabilizing the emotions, and facilitating access to untapped resources of the mind, aromatherapy promises to be an important transformational tool for psychotherapy, as well as for advancing spiritual awareness. As Cayce suggested, " . . . *there is the ability to make odors that will respond, and do respond, to certain individuals or groups; and many hundreds are responding to odors that produce the effect within their systems for activities that the psychoanalyst and the psychologist have long since discarded—much as they have the manner in which the Creative Forces or God may manifest in an individual!"* (274–10)

Aromatherapy plays an important role in the growing field of energy medicine. Applied with the right intent and purpose, aromatherapy might even become a tool for transcending the time and space limitations of the physical body by providing a direct link to that which is ever its builder—mind propelled by Spirit.

Healing with Light

Light and its visible manifestation, color, are all around us. If we consider the view of many of today's eminent physicists that matter is condensed light, then everything we see is an expression of light. It's not surprising then, that light and color have a measurable effect on our health and well–being. The focused use of light and color in our living environment can create moods and influence behavior. It can make us feel elated or pensive, happy or sad. It can trigger emotions of joy, anger, or tranquility, and promote health or disease. The Cayce readings say that *"all vibration, color, and color with radiation . . . is to set the vibrations in the body for body-forces . . . "* (3370-1) and *"the body mentally—and the body in its nerve reaction—would respond as quickly to color forces as it would to medicinal properties . . . "* (4501-1)

There are indeed modalities of holistic healing that use light and color therapeutically, as a primary healing tool or as an adjunct to other therapies. The ancient East Indian medical science of Ayurveda works with color to balance body energies that are out of harmony. In *Spiritual Nutrition and the Rainbow Diet*, author Gabriel Cousins, M.D., explains how foods of different colors influence the body via their effect on the chakras—the spiritual energy centers. Even if we disregard such esoteric principles and look to the strictly scientific recommendations of main-stream nutritionists, we are told that the healthiest foods are those that are strong in color—red, orange, and green—as they hold concentra-tions of important phytochemicals which have been shown to promote cellular rejuvenation and resistance to degenerative disease. However we view their effects, colors are indicators of powerful energies. Edgar Cayce writes in *Auras*: *"If colors are vibrations of spiritual forces, they should be able to help in healing our deepest and most subtle maladies. Together with music, which is a kindred spiritual force, they form a great hope for therapy of the future."* Cayce's prophetic powers were evident even in his own writings. It is fascinating to consider that several decades later, Dr. Jacob Liberman wrote a book documenting the therapeutic effects of light and color entitled *Light: Medicine of the Future.* The importance of natural sunlight for human health is one of the aspects emphasized in Dr. Liberman's book.

The Rejuvenating Effects of Sunlight.   On planet earth, in our corner of the universe, we depend on one single source of light for our survival: the sun. We know that without light from the sun, there would be no life on this planet. Sunlight sustains plants, animals, humans, and even the earth itself.

Yet in recent years, we've been inundated with information about the dangers of sunlight, and we have become conditioned to think that we must avoid the sun. By shunning sunlight and living a lifestyle that is primarily indoor-oriented, however, we miss out on all of the sun's wonderful life-giving properties. And subconsciously, we seem to have a growing awareness of our need for more sunlight. Who has not no-ticed the increasing popularity of decorative images of the sun and its ambassador, the sunflower, in recent years? Sunflowers have popped up on hats, T-shirts, oven mitts, coffee mugs, and tea towels; and their handcrafted counterparts pour sunny smiles from countless vases in malls and store windows.

As a universal symbol of the sun, the sunflower, and its recent ubiquitous appearance, may perhaps reflect a next step in humanity's awakening, on both a physical and a spiritual level. Deeply rooted in the earth, but always adjusting its angle to face the sun, the sunflower portrays the interconnectedness between life on earth and the light of the sun. Seen from a metaphysical perspective, the arts are a reflection of our collective unconscious, our common dreams seeking expression in the symbols and objects with which we surround ourselves. As the symbols of a dream are instrumental in conveying messages from the subconscious realms to our consciousness, so our current love affair with images of the sun may reflect a deeper knowledge stirring beneath the layers of our consciousness, and pointing to an aspect of our collective behavior requiring attention. Perhaps, by surrounding ourselves with arty renditions of the sun, we give expression to our yearning for its life–giving energy. Maybe it's time to put our acquired fear of the sun in its proper perspective.

Throughout history, the sun has been respected for its healing powers. In ancient Greece, physicians employed symptom–specific techniques of solar therapy by placing patients in specially constructed healing temples in the "sun city" of Heliopolis. Early in the twentieth century, prior to the discovery of antibiotic drugs, European physicians sent their tuberculosis patients to hospitals in the Swiss and Austrian Alps, where therapy consisted mainly of extended hours of sunbathing in the open air. The Cayce readings, too, suggested sunlight for TB and other ailments ranging from general debilitation to anemia and arthritis. Although one TB patient was told that *a good* sunburn all over *would be well for the body!"* (5554–2), the readings usually recommended sunshine in moderation, and warned against becoming overheated.

But who would dare go out in the sun these days? Reports of rapidly expanding holes in the earth's ozone layer are frightening enough to chase even the most committed of sun worshippers off the beach and into the "safe" fortresses of indoor swimming pools. While concern over the environmental practices that promote the destruction of the ozone layer is certainly warranted, we must not be misled into thinking that the sun is our enemy. Sunlight is not a killer. It is only when we lose touch with the natural instincts that guide us in our awareness of how to best interact with sun energy that we risk damage by excessive direct exposure, especially to the strong, midday sun, whose rays are particularly potent.

Enjoyed in moderation, and preferably during the early morning and mid- to late-afternoon hours, sunlight energizes, rejuvenates, and strengthens the body. Sunlight promotes good immune function and helps to fight infection, stimulate metabolism, and relieve insomnia and depression. In its physiological effects, sunlight is much like a nutrient which the body depends on for the smooth functioning of its glandular and metabolic systems. The Cayce readings acknowledge sunlight's role as an important co-factor in the proper activity of vitamins in the body. Reading 142–5 says: *"Keep the body under the sunlight, either directly or artificially, as much as possible. This for the strengthening of the blood supply and for the activity of the chrysalis, or of the forces as will build calcium in the system."*

Although excesses of ultraviolet radiation are potentially damaging, a certain amount of it is necessary for good health. Reading 566–2 says, *"It would be well for the body to be in the sunshine and air as much as possible through the seasons when the body may take on a great deal of the ultraviolet from the sun's rays."* UV rays, when absorbed by the skin, interact with chemicals in subcutaneous fatty tissue to produce vitamin D, which is necessary for the proper assimilation of calcium and other minerals from the diet. Research has shown that vitamin D synthesized from sunlight is physiologically superior to the form of the vitamin that is found in fortified foods and nutritional supplements.

Residents of northern latitudes frequently suffer from vitamin D deficiency, especially in the winter. Those who regularly use sunscreens are also at risk. Commercial sunscreens are promoted as the best protection against sun damage, next to complete sunlight avoidance. We are told to lather on sunscreen lotions with a high sun protection factor (SPF) whenever we venture outdoors. However, a growing number of scientists are concerned that sunscreens promote a false sense of security because they protect against sunburn but not against skin cancer. In fact, sunscreen use has been linked to higher skin cancer rates!

Most sunscreens work by blocking out ultraviolet B (UVB) rays, which cause reddening of sun-exposed skin and ultimately sunburn. Yet sunburn is the body's built-in alarm system—it tells us when we've had too much sun. When we turn off the alarm with a chemical sunscreen, our skin doesn't burn, but it still receives the longer ultraviolet A (UVA) rays, which are more dangerous. These rays are absorbed in the deep layers of the skin by melanocytes, which are involved in melanoma formation. They also depress the immune system and contribute to premature aging of skin.

UVB rays, on the other hand, help the skin make vitamin D. Preventing the skin from receiving UVB rays by applying sunscreen increases the risk of vitamin D deficiency. Older people are especially susceptible to this condition. An article in the April 28, 1998, issue of Tufts University *Health and Nutrition Letter* warns: *"People over 50 should not apply sunscreen as soon as they go outside—but wait 10 to 15 minutes,"* in addition to taking supplemental vitamin D. Low blood levels of vitamin D have also been associated with higher risk of breast and colon cancer and may accelerate the growth of melanoma.

If prolonged direct sun exposure is unavoidable, use a physical sunscreen which contains inert minerals such as titanium dioxide, zinc oxide, or talc. In contrast to chemical sunscreens, which absorb UVB rays, physical sunscreens reflect both types of ultraviolet rays away from the skin. Wearing light-colored clothing made from natural fiber will also reflect sunlight and help you stay cool.

Light Through the Eyes.   It is often said that the eyes are the windows of the soul. Pioneering research by photobiologist John N. Ott, Sc.D. (Hon.), has shown that they are also the doors through which light enters the body. A twist of fate that shattered the pair of glasses that Ott was wearing caused him to recognize the link between the sudden improvement in his arthritic condition and the natural sunlight that his eyes were able to absorb during the time he did not wear his glasses. From subsequent research findings, he concluded that the human body is a photosynthetic organism which depends on natural light for optimal health. Ott documented his findings in several excellent books, including *Health and Light: The Effects of Natural and Artificial Light on Man and Other Living Things*, and *Light, Radiation, and You: How to Stay Healthy*.

Light signals entering the eye serve a dual function: Some are utilized by photoreceptors on the retina for the process of vision, while others travel to the brain, where they are interpreted by the hypothalamus. The hypothalamus regulates the function of the autonomic nervous system and also initiates various hormonal activities via the pituitary gland. It controls the release of the hormone melatonin by the pineal gland in response to environmental darkness and therefore is also involved in regulating the body's sleep/wake cycle. Disruptions of this cycle have been shown to be implicated in a number of health problems. For instance, a study conducted in 2001 at the Fred Hutchinson Cancer Research Center in Seattle, Washington, showed that women who are persistently exposed to light at night—whether because they work the nightshift, suffer from insomnia, or are exposed to light in their bedrooms—have an increased risk of developing breast cancer. Researchers speculate that the reason may be that when normal melatonin cycles are interrupted, the production of estrogen from the ovaries is higher, and this may contribute to the women's higher breast cancer risk.

Similarly, a sustained shortage of natural full-spectrum light waves during the day results in imbalances of the nervous and endocrine systems, producing symptoms which range from reduced metabolism and sleep disturbances to immune deficiencies. Residents of the northern latitudes are all too familiar with the winter blues, manifesting as fatigue, lethargy, irritability, or downright depression. In extreme cases, individuals suffering from Seasonal Affective Disorder (SAD) become severely dysfunctional and even suicidal. An effective therapy for people afflicted with SAD is stimulation of the eyes with full-spectrum light, including ultraviolet.

But what about the various reports of UV radiation causing cataracts and skin cancer? In *Light: Medicine of the Future*, optometrist Jacob Liberman explains that much of the concern over ultraviolet rays is based on experiments on monkeys. Strong light containing high levels of UV radiation was beamed into the tranquilized animals' forcibly opened eyes for sixteen minutes. Dr. Liberman says that such concentrated exposure would never happen in real life, since the monkey's pupils and eyelids would contract and close to protect the eye. The retinal damage that these monkeys sustained is often cited in claiming that UV light also causes cataracts.

According to findings by John Ott, some low–level UV radiation is essential for the maintenance of good vision, as it promotes mitosis of the pigment epithelial tissue, located just behind the retina. On a bright, sunny day, most people experience an improvement in visual acuity. Other beneficial effects of UV light include improvement of heart function, reduction of cholesterol levels, and lowering of blood pressure.

Cayce reading 349–22 also points to the importance of absorbing some UV light: *"Also we would have rest periods, and keep in the sunshine as much as practical; that there may be the absorption of the ultraviolet activities through the system itself. These are better gained or attained from the exercises in the sunshine than in any other form."*

As with everything in life, moderation is the key. Even before the destruction of the ozone layer became a concern, common sense was called for when going out in the sun. Sunbathing is best enjoyed during the early morning and late afternoon hours, and it is best to remain in the shade on a hot summer day. The full spectrum of beneficial light rays can reach the body even in the shade. Dr. Liberman recommends spending at least half an hour outdoors daily, preferably in the early morning. Since most contact and prescription lenses, as well as dark sunglasses, block out a portion of the light spectrum, he suggests removing them during that time to improve vision and general health.

Meir Schneider, Ph.D., is author and coauthor respectively of two books on self–healing and founder of the School for Self–Healing in San Francisco, California. He cured himself of congenital blindness through the intensive and consistent application of vision exercises. Schneider recommends a technique called "sunning" for vision improvement. With your eyes closed, stand erect, facing the sun, and slowly turn the head from side to side several times. This allows sunlight to alternately stimulate different photoreceptors on the surface of the retina. It is important to never look directly at the sun. A wide–brimmed hat to protect the eyes and face from direct sunlight is preferable to sunglasses.

With sunlight as with all things, moderation is the key. Cayce's advice that *"Sunshine is always beneficial to a body, if it is not overdone,"* (2072–9) could well serve as a good guideline in helping us to know when and how to interact with the sun for optimal health and well–being. Our mental, emotional, and spiritual health is inextricably connected with the health of our bodies, as long as we dwell in them. As we seek to awaken spiritually, we must open ourselves to the physical manifestation of Spirit in the earth plane: light energy. We are beings of light, and as such, we cannot separate ourselves from the source that fuels our bodies, the sun.

Even as the great healing potential of sunlight goes largely unrecognized in medical circles today, there were those who doubted it in Cayce's time. However, the readings say that it will ultimately become evident on its own strength: " . . . *there is the tendency of individuals in the profession that belittle the value of light or sunlight; yet . . . the effectiveness of the light will demonstrate in itself its value, even as common sense shows the valuation of sunlight to every form of vegetation, from the lowest to the highest."* (165–12)

Sound as Healer

In our industrialized world, noise is a major contributor to ill health. Those of us who live in cities know that "noise pollution" is just as real as air pollution. Exposure to constant noise wears down the nervous system and causes irritability, headaches, and even cardiovascular problems. In noisy urban areas, the use of tranquilizers is considerably higher than average. An increasing percentage of employee absenteeism, caused by conditions ranging from fatigue to mental stress and depression, can be directly attributed to noise. A study reported in the October 2000 issue of the *Journal of Applied Psychology* found that those who work in noisy open–office environments showed increased levels of the stress hormone epinephrine. Research conducted at the University of Gavle in Sweden in 2002 showed that children living near airports, who were exposed to the noise that accompanies the take–off and landing of airplanes on a regular basis, had poorer short– and long-term memory, as well as poorer speech perception and reading abilities, than children not exposed to such noise.

Silence, harmonious music, and the sounds of nature are the perfect antidote to stressful conditions caused by a noisy environment. As Cayce reading 1334–1 says, " . . . *sounds, music and colors may have much to do with creating the proper vibrations about individuals that are mentally unbalanced, physically deficient or ill in body and mind . . .* " Another reading says that certain types of music can indeed help to bring a person out of a state of despondency: *"And whenever there are the periods of depression, or the feeling low or forsaken, play music; especially stringed instruments of every nature. These will enable the entity to span that gulf as between pessimism and optimism."* (1804-1)

The use of sound therapy dates back to ancient times. Even Pythagoras is said to have taught that certain rhythms and melodies have a medicinal effect on the body. Indigenous people worldwide use sound in a ceremonial manner. Shamanic rituals especially work with sound techniques such as drumming to invoke a therapeutic effect. Religious ceremonies, throughout the ages, have relied on ritualistic song and chanting to facilitate spiritual attunement. The Cayce readings recommend that we *"Learn more of music . . . Get the harmony and peace that such brings. And know its source, that must arise in self."* (3084-1)

Today, even mainstream medicine is showing considerable interest in the ability of sound to soothe and heal. In 2001, researchers at John Hopkins University in Baltimore, Maryland, found that natural sounds and images could improve pain control and reduce anxiety levels in patients who were undergoing a diagnostic exam for lung disease that is associated with a certain amount of discomfort. In the same year, a study conducted at the State University of New York at Buffalo discovered that music helped reduce the stress experience by elderly patients undergoing outpatient eye surgery. The patients were allowed to choose the specific music that they wanted to hear during the surgery. The control group was not given this option. On the morning of the surgery, all patients' blood pressure rose in anticipation of the procedure. However, in the test group, blood pressure returned to normal within five minutes of the patients' hearing the music.

The ability of harmonious music to lower blood pressure was also observed in an earlier study conducted in 2000 at Kaleida Health-Millard Fillmore Hospital in Buffalo, New York. In this study, test subjects who had normal blood pressure readings were subjected to a task that caused mental stress, resulting in a rise in blood pressure. It was noted that afterwards, blood pressure in the test subjects who listened to classical music or nature sounds returned to normal in less time than the control group—in an average of 2.9 and 3.0 minutes respectively, vs. the norm of 3.7 minutes.

In 2002, researchers at the General Hospital of Salzburg, Austria, found that daily listening to music while being given instructions on using relaxation imagery helped patients with chronic low back pain after surgery for a herniated disk to reduce pain and sleep disturbances. The researchers concluded that soft or classical music, working on the autonomic nervous system, helped to promote muscle relaxation and dissolve tension, thus aiding in pain management.

Research done in 2001 at Orebro Medical Center Hospital in Sweden also suggests that soothing music and encouraging words played to patients who are under anesthesia may help ease their recovery following the surgery. It appears that even though patients who are under general anesthesia are unconscious, there is an awareness (the researchers say it is "the brain") that records everything that happens during the surgery. Comments and remarks made by doctors and nurses during the surgery are nevertheless "heard" by the patient, who sometimes responds with anxiety, illness, or dissatisfaction after the procedure. The study suggests that when soothing music or nature sounds such as ocean waves are played to patients during the surgery, there may be less pain and fatigue after the procedure, and patients recover more quickly.

This study demonstrates the powerful ability of music to soothe and relax, but it also confirms what Edgar Cayce, as well as other metaphysically oriented teachers, have said about the nature of human consciousness—that the subconscious records and responds to sounds played and to "suggestions" given during the time that consciousness is suspended, through general anesthesia or presleep and other sleep-like states.

The potential for using music to facilitate healing is enormous. The Cayce readings say, *"Do get the note vibrations in music to which the body will respond and continue to interest the body in same whenever the treatments are given."* (3401–1) and *"Keep about the body . . . music that is of harmony—as of the Spring Song, the Blue Danube and that character of music, with either the stringed instruments or the organ. These are the vibrations that will set again near normalcy—yea, normalcy, mentally and physically . . . "* (2712–1)

What is it that makes music and sound such a powerful healer or destroyer? A study published in the September 25 issue of the *Proceed-*

ings of the National Academy of Sciences showed that music that solicits a strong emotional response in people activated the brain's reward and emotion centers—the same areas that are "turned on" when stimulated by food, sex, and addictive substances such as alcohol and nicotine. Music thus affects people at the very depth of their being. The Cayce readings say that music is "of the soul," and that *"Music is as . . . a destructive or creative force, dependent upon that to which it appeals in the influence of individuals."* (3509–1) In *The Secret Music of the Soul*, author Patrick Bernhardt says: *"The basic nature of the music we listen to invariably leaves its imprint on our mores, actions and patterns of behaviour."*

May our prayer be that, individually and as a society, we become more conscious in our selection of the music and the sounds that we allow ourselves and our children to hear, so that we may be healed instead of sickened, and that ultimately, we may join with the angels in song for the glory of God. Let us remember Cayce reading 5401–1, which says, *"For music is of the soul, and one may become mind and soul-sick for music, or soul and mind-sick from certain kinds of music."*

Homeopathy

Homeopathy has become an increasingly popular method for the treatment of common ailments. I had researched homeopathy for a number of years before experiencing its enormous healing potential firsthand when suffering from an excruciating toothache. My dentist had replaced a very large filling in a lower–jaw molar. For several days after the procedure, the discomfort and soreness remained until it became a throbbing toothache that was so painful that I could hardly breathe. Warm drinks or foods aggravated the pain. It was Friday afternoon and the dentist's office was closed. Finally, a friend handed me a homeopathic remedy for nerve pain, *hypericum*, in a 30C dilution. Within thirty seconds of taking the remedy, the pain vanished and did not return until months later, at which time another dentist whom I consulted explained that the filling was just too deep and the tooth needed a root canal.

A short time later, my husband had a similar experience with an infected tooth that began bothering him one afternoon. After a few hours, the only way he could cope with the pain was by continuously cooling down the tooth and surrounding area with sips of cold water. An after-hours phone call to the dentist, who had training in homeopathy, resulted in an extensive question–and–answer period, during which the dentist tried to determine the exact nature of the pain. When the dentist was satisfied that he had a complete picture of the symptoms, he recommended a 30C solution of the homeopathic remedy *camomila*, which we happened to have in our natural remedies cabinet from the time that our son was teething. The remedy made the pain disappear instantly. My husband went to the dentist the following morning to have the tooth treated, but the homeopathic remedy had made it possible for him to go to bed that night and get a pain–free night's sleep.

Both these stories involve dental problems, but that's just a coincidence. Homeopathic remedies can be used for any ailment at all. Because they are easy to administer and virtually free of side effects, they are particularly popular in the treatment of common children's ailments.

In homeopathy, a substance or an agent that can cause specific symptoms in healthy people is used to stimulate the body's immune system to defend itself against that agent. The Greek roots of the word homeopathy are *homoios*, meaning same, and *pathos*, meaning the occurrence of suffering. Samuel Hahnemann, a nineteenth–century German physician who pioneered the development of contemporary homeopathic medicine, coined the Latin phrase *"similia similibus curantur"*—like cures like. The principle behind this is similar to vaccination, except that in the case of homeopathy, the substance that is used is diluted to such an extent that, ultimately, not a trace of the actual substance remains, but that only an imprint of its energy is present in the medium—usually lactose pellets or water. Homeopathic remedies are "potentized," using an alcohol solution, through vigorous shaking called *succussion*. A process referred to as *trituration* is used to potentize substances that are naturally insoluble in alcohol. By grinding such substances as mercury, calcium carbonate, or sulphur, with powdered sugar or milk, they can ultimately be dissolved in alcohol. Homeopathy holds that the more diluted the remedy is, the stronger its effects are.

Because most homeopathic remedies contain none of the original substance, but only an energy imprint, mainstream medicine has, for the most part, regarded homeopathy as quackery. In recent years, however, several research trials have validated the effects of homeopathy. A study published in the August 19, 2000, issue of the *British Medical Journal* demonstrated that treating patients who suffered from perennial hay fever with homeopathic remedies was significantly more effective than a placebo (inactive medication). This study was conducted under strict observance of scientific standards at the Glasgow Homeopathic Hospital.

How can a remedy in extremely high dilutions possibly show such an effect? In the early 1990s, a small team of French scientists led by Jacques Benveniste made an amazing discovery that offers an explanation for why homeopathic preparations are effective in high dilutions which lack any detectable molecules of the originally dissolved substance. Known as the hypothesis of water, this theory addresses the capacity of water to somehow organize in a stable manner and thereby acquire the ability to store and play back information obtained from other molecules.

In his book *The Memory of Water*, author Michael Schiff reports that Jacques Benveniste also theorizes that water's apparent ability to transport chemical information without any transfer of the corresponding molecules might have something to do with electromagnetic fields. The idea seems to be substantiated by the finding that a low-frequency alternating magnetic field appears to be capable of erasing the memory. The book claims that to date, still no one knows precisely how the molecular organization of water could permit the storage and playback of chemical information, and mainstream science has largely ignored and even ridiculed Benveniste's research experiments, repeatedly carried out with rigorous scrutiny and under strict observance of all scientific rules and guidelines.

Homeopathic remedies are prepared from a variety of materials, including plant tissue, mineral substances, common allergens such as grass pollen, and even animal substances and diseased tissue. One animal-tissue-based homeopathic remedy that was recommended in several Cayce readings for the treatment of phlebitis and edema is the juice from the cimex lectularius, commonly known as "bedbug." A tincture prepared from ragweed, although not technically a homeopathic remedy, was recommended by Cayce as a liver tonic and preventive remedy for seasonal ragweed allergies. In homeopathy, it is important to identify the exact right remedy for a specific condition. Unless this criteria is met, the homeopathic remedy will be ineffective. At best, an inappropriate homeopathic remedy does no harm because the body does not respond to a remedy that is not required. It takes much training and great skill to identify the proper homeopathic remedy, not only for a specific condition, but also for the constitution of the patient. There are many excellent books available that provide information on the types of remedies to be used for certain pathologies. Longstanding conditions or those that do not seem to respond to over-the-counter homeopathic remedies may require the expertise of a qualified homeopathic practitioner.

The Radial Appliance and Wet Cell Battery

A discussion of energy medicine in the context of the Cayce readings would not be complete without a description of two electrotherapeutic devices frequently recommended by Cayce: the radial appliance and the wet cell battery. I am indebted to Dr. Dudley Delany, author of *The Edgar Cayce Way of Overcoming Multiple Sclerosis: Vibratory Medicine* (available online at http://members.tripod.com/~dudley_delany/index-70.html and in hard cover through the A.R.E. Bookstore at 757-428-3588, ext. 7231), for kindly providing the following information pertaining to these devices:

> *The radial appliance (also referred to as the impedance device, the radio-active appliance, and the dry cell) was recommended in over nine hundred readings for such conditions as deafness, debilitation, hypertension, leukemia, migraine, nervous tension, obesity, poor circulation, psoriasis, sterility, tic douloureux, and tuberculosis.*
>
> *It consists of a small metal container containing two rectangular steel rods separated by glass plates and surrounded on four sides by carbon. This steel-glass-carbon "sandwich" is wrapped in tape and immersed in charcoal particles. Each steel rod attaches to a terminal on the outside of the appliance. Wires plug into the terminals that*

lead to small nickel electrodes. Placement of these electrodes normally involves the wrists and ankles.

The appliance is activated by partial immersion in ice water twenty minutes before attachment of the electrodes to the body. A typical session on the device usually lasts between thirty minutes to an hour.

The appliance does not generate any measurable electricity of its own. Instead, it induces and modulates the flow of a naturally occurring form of electricity produced by the body itself.

The primary purpose of the radial appliance is to promote relaxation, improve circulation, and balance the body mentally, physically, and spiritually.

The wet cell battery (also known as the wet cell appliance) was recommended in about 975 readings for the treatment of such conditions as alcoholism, Alzheimer's disease, amyotrophic lateral sclerosis, cancer, color blindness, Down's syndrome, Parkinson's disease, major depression, muscular dystrophy, multiple sclerosis, Parkinson's disease, polio, rheumatoid arthritis, schizophrenia, scleroderma, spinal cord injury, and stroke.

It consists of a nonmetallic container about the size of a car battery in which two metal rods (one made of copper and the other of nickel) are suspended in an electrolytic solution containing distilled water, copper sulfate, sulfuric acid, zinc, and willow charcoal.

On top of each pole is a terminal. The wet cell generates a very small, normally imperceptible current that, in electrical terms, causes the terminal attached to the copper pole to become positive and the one attached to the nickel pole to become negative.

The wire that plugs into the positive terminal attaches to a small copper electrode that is most often placed at various points along the spine. The wire that plugs into the negative terminal routes the electricity through a small jar in which various medicinal agents can be placed, and then on to a larger nickel electrode which is usually placed just above and to the right of the navel.

The wiring is attached to the wet cell twenty minutes before use, and sessions generally last thirty minutes.

By far the most frequently recommended medicinal agent was a very dilute solution of gold chloride. The readings stated that such a *medium would help rejuvenate any organ that was "delinquent" in its action.*

The primary purpose of the wet cell battery is to introduce into the body the vibratory energy of the medicinal agent placed in the solution jar. When properly done, this simple procedure has far reaching consequences and ramifications in terms of restoring proper functioning to bodily tissues, organs, and systems. In this writer's opinion, it has the potential for revolutionizing the treatment of diseases and conditions currently thought to be hopeless and incurable.

Research using the appliances, although small-scale, has tended to confirm their utility, and there presently exists numerous anecdotal accounts of their effectiveness.

For more information about these two devices, the interested reader is referred to an excellent book by David McMillin, M.A., and Douglas G. Richards, Ph.D., The Radial Appliance and the Wet Cell Battery. *For ordering information, call the A.R.E. Bookstore at 757-428-3588, ext. 7231. That same number may also be used to purchase the appliances and their various accessories.*

Baar Products, the official worldwide supplier of Edgar Cayce health care products, manufactures both the Radio–Active Appliance, which they call the Radiac®, and the Wet Cell Battery. In 1987, the Fetzer Energy Medicine Research Institute launched a double–blind scientific study on the Radiac. The study results show that the Radiac had a measurable effect on the human neuroendocrine system, promoting stress reduction and relaxation indicated by better coordination of the circulatory system. The study details are published in *The Radiac Book*, which can be obtained from Baar Products through their Web site, www.baar.com, or by calling 610–873–4591 or 1–800–269–2502.

Healing the Mind—
And Using the Mind to Heal

"... Think health, bring health ... "   Edgar Cayce reading 900-254

MORE THAN 450 million people worldwide suffer from some kind of mental or neurological disorder, according to the World Health Organization. Based on information gathered from 191 member states, WHO estimates that 120 million people worldwide have clinical depression, 50 million have epilepsy, 37 million suffer from Alzheimer's disease, and 24 million from schizophrenia. WHO further says that 25 percent of the world's population will suffer from one or more mental disorders at some point in their lives.

Looking at these figures, one can't help but wonder about the cause of such problems—what is it that's driving us insane and causing us to lose hope? Does mental illness strike at random, like a bolt of lightning out of the blue? Or is genetic predisposition the determining influence, or the process of aging, or perhaps the environment? Can we accept the responsibility that our mental health is also influenced by our lifestyle, by our choice of foods, our choice of friends and leisure activities, by our work—even by the thoughts we think?

The Cayce readings leave no doubt that "... *thoughts* are *things, and as their currents run must bring their own seed.*" (288–29) We are also told what happens to the mind when we don't pay attention and direct our thoughts in a hopeful and positive way: "... *for unless there is the expectancy, unless there is hope ... [the mind's] outlook becomes a drag, a drug on the hands of one that is being attacked from within ... by the dis-eases of a physical body.*" (572–5) Mental and physical health go hand in hand and will either lift each other up, or drag each other down.

So where do we start if we want to prevent and heal mental disorders, or mental decline as we age? An examination of the lifestyle factors that appear to either promote or ward off illnesses such as depression, Alzheimer's, and impaired mental performance or memory loss, can provide clues as to how we might avoid certain risk factors and implement a lifestyle that promotes mental and physical fitness in good measure.

Staying Active Keeps the Mind Healthy

Regular exercise benefits not only physical health but also keeps our minds sharp as we age. A study published in the July 23, 2001, issue of the journal *Archives of Internal Medicine* showed that among women aged sixty-five and older, those who were the most physically active at the beginning of the study were least likely to experience a decline in mental function during the next six to eight years. The exercise need not be strenuous—even moderate activity is effective. And it stands to reason that the benefits would not be exclusive to older people; if exercise can promote mental acuity in an older person, then it would do the same for an individual at any age. Previous research has also shown that those who exercise regularly live longer than those who don't.

Exercise stimulates circulation, so that nutrients are readily transported to the cells, including brain cells. Better circulation to the brain promotes greater mental clarity. Exercise also encourages the release of beta-endorphins—brain chemicals with analgesic properties that produce a feeling of relaxation and well-being. As we have seen in chapter 5, Edgar Cayce's head-and-neck exercises are one of the best ways for improving circulation to the brain.

Keeping the mind active is in itself a way of preserving mental powers. A study done at Columbia University in New York in 2001 found that leisure activities such as reading, going to the movies, or visiting with friends and relatives could lower the risk of developing dementia. Other research, published in the February 28, 2002, issue of the journal *Neuron*, suggests that certain types of rehabilitation and brain training exercises can strengthen memory skills. This study provides evidence that memory loss is not, as previously thought, due to the destruction of brain cells in the area of the prefrontal cortex region, the part of the brain responsible for memories. Rather, it is a question of gradually reduced activity in the prefrontal cortex, which can be increased using certain memory strategies and training exercises. Earlier research at the Central Arkansas Veterans Healthcare System in Little Rock had also shown that brain volume does not stop expanding after age twenty, as was commonly believed, but that it continues to increase until the mid- to late-forties. And just as exercise builds muscle, continued stimulation to the brain and mental challenges can promote brain growth. Preliminary animal research has even shown that the brain is capable of repairing itself and growing new cells after an injury. More research is required in this area, but in the meantime, we know that by keeping the mind active and adequately challenged, we can preserve the health of the vehicle that the mind uses to function—the brain.

Pathological conditions also have an influence on memory. Research conducted at the University of Pittsburgh and Western Psychiatric Institute showed that high blood pressure impaired blood flow to the brain parts associated with memory, causing loss of working memory in these patients. A study published in the December 2000 issue of *Annals of Neurology* also demonstrated that long-term changes in diastolic blood pressure—the second reading done when measuring blood pressure—may be linked to higher risk of dementia in the elderly. Keeping blood pressure under control is therefore just as important for good mental health as it is for physical health.

So, keeping healthy and staying active both physically and mentally can do wonders to preserve good mental function at any age. Cayce reading 1010-4 holds good advice in this regard that's easy to remember: *"Keep the mind active and the body in motion . . . "*

Heal the Mind—Get a Handle on Stress

Mental imbalances, including memory loss, anxiety, and depression, can have many causes, but a major factor at the root of these conditions and many other modern ills is often stress. Our hectic schedules and the myriad of activities we're involved in on a daily basis, as well as a constant barrage of sensory stimulation, wreak havoc with the nervous system and exhaust us mentally and physically. The mind/body connection is highly evident when we consider the effects of mental and emotional stress. Stress weakens immune response and predisposes us to degenerative disease. We can't always avoid stress, but we can learn to change the ways in which we respond to the stressors in our lives. Poor stress response triggers a biochemical reaction in the body that impacts the nervous system as well as organ function. Research has shown that patients with psychotic illness are more affected by stressful events than healthy individuals. According to a study published in the August 2001 issue of *Stroke: Journal of the American Heart Association*, the way in which an individual handles stress can be associated with the incidence of stroke. The cardiovascular system's reaction to stress has been shown to influence the development of artery disease and other factors that affect stroke risk. Stress–induced blood pressure increases have also been linked to stroke. Research reported in the May 27, 2000, issue of the *British Medical Journal* found that job stress had measurable effects on mental and physical health. Among a group of nurses, those whose jobs were the most demanding were more likely to report symptoms of anxiety and depression. Chronic stress has also been shown to increase the risk of cervical neoplasia—the precursor to cervical cancer—according to research conducted at the University of South Carolina in Columbia.

So we need to reduce stress in our lives, or at least change the ways in which we habitually respond to stressful situations. Getting enough rest and regular breaks from the daily routine helps to keep a healthy perspective on stressful events. Spending time outdoors, close to nature, helps to soothe the nervous system and regain a more peaceful and positive mental outlook. Healing the mind and healing the body really do go hand in hand. The Cayce readings say: *"Have more time for the outdoors, and for the relaxation of the body. Do not have too great a stress upon the system."* (528–13) and *"The body needs the rest, outdoors, oxygen, carbons, those elements that will meet the needs of the system and produce the resistive forces in the body."* (4383–3)

Herbal remedies are also effective to help guard against the impact of stress. A popular herb for relieving stress and anxiety is valerian root. Throughout Europe, valerian is known as a nonaddictive alternative to pharmaceutical nerve relaxants. Research in recent years has confirmed valerian's ability to gently sedate the central nervous system. Valerian tincture was recommended in several Cayce readings.

As we have seen in chapter 5, St. John's wort has been shown in clinical studies to relieve the anxiety and depression often associated with stress. It does so without the unpleasant side effects that are common with pharmaceutical antidepressants.

Another excellent natural relaxant that was discussed in the aromatherapy section of chapter 5 is lavender, whose essential oil has a soothing effect on the nervous system through its action, via the olfactory bulb, on the brain's limbic system and the hypothalamus gland. Lavender was frequently recommended in the Cayce readings.

Homeopathic remedies are also helpful in relieving fatigue and anxiety that often result from stress. *Gelsemium* helps mental confusion and an overall feeling of weakness from nervous exhaustion. *Arsenicum album* and *carbo vegetabilis* help with restlessness and excessive nervousness causing the hands and feet to become cold and painful.

The importance of sleep was discussed in chapter 4. According to research done at the National University of Singapore, sleep deprivation, especially on an ongoing basis, causes the release of hormones which increase sleepiness. Those who have to force themselves to stay awake despite such sleepiness are put under considerable psychological stress. The researchers concluded that sleep is not negotiable, but is a biological imperative. Loss of sleep extracts a major toll in terms of our health and mental capacity. As the Cayce readings say, *"Sleep is a sense, as we have given . . . and is that needed for the physical body to recuperate, or to draw from the mental and spiritual powers or forces that are held as the ideals of the body."*

(2067-3) Getting enough sleep must be a priority in our stress control program if we want to enjoy good physical and mental health.

One of the best methods for quickly overcoming feelings of stress is deep breathing. When we are nervous or upset, breathing becomes shallow, reducing oxygen supply in the body and aggravating fatigue and anxiety. Concentrating on breathing slowly and deeply for a few minutes, several times a day, can help us feel relaxed, energized, and invigorated. Edgar Cayce said, *"Rest sufficiently but keep in the open as much as possible, especially in the sunshine. Breathe deep!"* (1548-1) For more information on the benefits of deep breathing, see the section on the benefits of exercising outdoors in chapter 4.

Food and Mood—the Mind/Body Connection

The foods we eat have a significant influence on brain function and therefore on mental performance. The brain's main source of fuel is glucose (blood sugar), an end product of carbohydrate metabolism, which is used by the cells for energy. Glucose is fed to the brain via the bloodstream. Fluctuations in glucose levels affect brain chemistry and can produce anxiety, irritability, and confusion. Dr. Abram Hoffer, a pioneer in nutrition–oriented psychiatry, has found that some 60 percent of schizophrenics have severe hypoglycemia (low blood sugar).

The elimination of white sugar and refined carbohydrates from the diet is the most important step in the prevention and treatment of glucose imbalances. Refined carbohydrates, such as white sugar, white flour, white rice, and pasta made with refined grains, are best avoided. They are converted to glucose rapidly, resulting in excessive blood sugar levels. The liver is forced to speed up glucose metabolism until blood sugar levels drop off. While refined sugar products provide quick spurts of energy, they tend to produce a yo-yo effect in blood sugar levels. This results in mood swings, disrupted attention span, and inability to concentrate.

Unrefined complex carbohydrates, such as whole grain products, legumes, carrots, and Jerusalem artichokes, are much better brain food choices. Their conversion to glucose takes place gradually, ensuring a constant and steady supply of energy. It is important, however, to balance starchy foods with lighter, green vegetables which supply blood–building minerals, powerful antioxidants, and other health–promoting phytochemicals.

Another important reason for choosing whole grains rather than their refined counterparts is the full range of amino acids, vitamins, and trace minerals in the germ and outer layers of the grain. In refined foods, these are scraped off during the milling process. Amino acids are the building blocks of protein in the body and are essential for the production of neurotransmitters, the chemicals involved in the electronic transmission of nerve impulses across nerve synapses in the brain. Foods rich in high–quality amino acids promote mental alertness and increased energy levels and should be consumed regularly throughout the day. Good dietary sources of amino acids are organic meats, fish, and eggs, as well as combinations of whole grains, legumes, and nuts and seeds.

A study published in the August 2001 issue of the journal *Neuropsychopharmacology* showed that the consumption of the essential amino acid tryptophan helped people to be more self–confident. Tryptophan is the precursor to the brain chemical serotonin, a neurotransmitter which promotes relaxation and calmness. Low serotonin levels have been associated with depression, impulsivity, and aggressive behavior. Study subjects who took three grams of tryptophan daily were more sure of themselves and were less quarrelsome than the control group that was taking an inactive placebo. Good sources of tryptophan include dairy products and turkey meat. Carbohydrate–rich foods also boost serotonin production. It is best, however, to source these carbohydrates from whole grains and vegetables, which provide better long–term energy support than refined starches and sweets.

The mineral chromium helps to regulate blood–sugar levels and can thus contribute to the prevention of emotional ups and downs. An excellent food source of chromium is brewer's yeast, which also supplies vitamins of the B complex, known as the "stress vitamins." These nutrients are essential for the healthy functioning of the brain and entire nervous system. A chronic deficiency in one or more B vitamins can produce symptoms such as mental confusion, memory loss, aggressiveness, 'depression, and hysteria. A vitamin B6 deficiency, in particular, is associated with emotional disorders. This is because B6 plays an important role in the production of the brain chemicals serotonin and dopamine, neurotransmitters which regulate nerve function, mood, memory, and sleep. Niacin, another member of the B complex, also plays an important role in maintaining mental health. Dr. Hoffer successfully treated cases of mild schizophrenia with high doses of niacin, a member of the B complex. Among the B–vitamin sources favored by Cayce are steel-cut oats, whole grains, and yellow–colored vegetables and fruits. The B vitamins are also present in green leafy vegetables, legumes, eggs, and dairy products. In supplement form, B vitamins are best taken combined in a well–balanced, low–potency B–complex formula, as they function synergistically.

Also important for brain function is natural vitamin E (d–alpha tocopherol), which preserves cellular DNA repair function and fights free radicals, which cause tissue degeneration and destruction of brain cells. Vitamin E promotes blood circulation to the brain and other tissues. Wheat germ oil is especially high in this vitamin. Make sure it is freshly pressed—stored wheat germ oil is prone to rancidity. Other good sources of vitamin E are almonds, walnuts, cashews, butter, and eggs.

Vitamin C (ascorbic acid) promotes tissue regeneration and strengthens blood vessels. When taken together with bioflavonoids such as quercetin, rutin, and hesperidin, vitamin C blocks the spontaneous oxidation reactions leading to the creation of free radicals which promote tissue degeneration and destruction of brain cells. Vitamin C and bioflavonoids are found in many fresh vegetables and fruit, particularly citrus fruit. A study reported in the March 2000 issue of *Neurology* found that elderly men who took supplements of vitamin C and E at least once a week for several years were protected from dementia and actually showed improvement in cognitive function, including memory capacity, creativity, and mental acuity. The researchers concluded that vitamin C and E supplements may protect against dementia and improve cognitive function later in life.

A deficiency of calcium and magnesium in the body can disrupt the transmission of nerve impulses, promoting a feeling of edginess and irritability. Good dietary sources of these important minerals are dark-green leafy vegetables, almonds, and sea vegetables. Calcium is also

derived from egg yolks, dairy products, sesame seeds, carrots, and tur-
nips, as well as from chewing the soft ends of chicken bones, a source
often recommended by Cayce. Mummy food, so called because the
recipe was given to Edgar Cayce in a dream by an Egyptian mummy,
provides calcium and magnesium in an optimal ratio (2:1). Mummy
food is a mixture of equal parts dates and figs, cooked with cornmeal
and water to a smooth consistency. The readings say that mummy food,
taken with milk, could be considered *"almost a spiritual food . . . "* (275–45).
The significant amounts of calcium and magnesium, as well as B vitamins, which mummy food provides, help to relax the nervous system
and promote mental and emotional tranquility, important attributes of
spiritual poise.

Breakfast Sets the Mood. The effect of a single meal on the
mood of the day is often underestimated. Take a typical weekday breakfast of fruit juice, coffee, toast, and jam. High in sugar, starch, and caffeine, it provides just enough quick energy to help fight one's way
through rush-hour traffic. By the time many folks get to work, blood
sugar levels have dropped and they feel edgy or tired and need another
caffeine fix. But adding a protein food, such as free-range eggs or cot-
tage cheese to the above breakfast, would slow down sugar metabolism
and provide longer-lasting energy.

A nutritious breakfast helps to ensure mood stability and mental
alertness throughout the day. A study reported in the November 2001
issue of the *American Journal of Clinical Nutrition*, showed that eating breakfast improved memory performance in test subjects. In your choice of
foods, emphasize whole foods that release glucose slowly. High-quality
proteins and natural fats in moderation slow down food absorption
and help stabilize energy. Chewing foods well is important. The Cayce
readings frequently emphasize the importance of chewing for proper
digestion and assimilation. Research done at the Gifu University School
of Medicine in Japan also showed that the act of chewing itself promotes better memory performance. The researchers found that the
chewing movements of the jaws signal the hippocampus areas of the
brain, which is critical for learning. Other researchers in the U.K. believe
that chewing may improve memory by reducing stress. Whatever the

specific mechanism may be, this study shows that we would do well to remember Edgar Cayce's advice:

> *Chew any mouthful of food at least fourteen times. Even in drinking water,* chew *it—or masticate it at least three or four times. That is, sip it—let the activity of the glands in the mouth mingle well with the water; not gulping it but sipping it gently.*   595-1

The Coffee Question.   For many people, a cup of coffee in the morning is a part of their breakfast they would not like to give up. Research done at the University of Arizona in Tucson suggests that coffee helps to improve memory in older adults. The study, published in the January 2002 issue of *Psychological Science*, showed that older adults who drank a twelve-ounce cup of regular coffee before taking a memory test performed better than those who drank decaffeinated coffee. Other research has shown that coffee drinkers face a lower risk of developing Parkinson's disease, a neurological disease that produces symptoms such as tremor, loss of facial expression, and difficulties with balance and walking. Yet other studies shed a more negative light on America's favorite morning drink, suggesting that drinking coffee may put healthy individuals at risk for decreased insulin sensitivity, a precursor to diabetes. The Cayce readings frequently refer to coffee as having food value, saying that coffee is *"preferable to many stimulants that may be taken . . . "* (294–86) However, it was also emphasized that coffee should be taken black, without milk or cream, and with little or no sugar: *"Coffee, taken properly, is a food; that is,* without *cream or milk."* (303–2) and *"Coffee may be taken in moderation if desired, provided it is taken* without *milk or cream, using* very *little sugar!"* (2315–1) As in all things, moderation is emphasized because caffeine, taken in excess, can stimulate the nervous system to such an extent that the coffee drinker experiences the jitters, nervousness, and anxiety.

The Endocrine Connection

Hormonal fluctuations can also affect brain function, mental performance, and the way in which we view each other and the world around us. It is no secret that menstruation, pregnancy, childbirth, and meno-pause are often accompanied by a change in mental outlook and symp-toms of emotional instability ranging from mild to severe. The Cayce readings emphasize that endocrine imbalances could play a major role in depression, precipitated by failure of the glands to adequately nour-ish the cells of the nervous system. A natural whole foods diet, along with appropriate nutritional supplements, can help to remedy such imbalances.

Among the most important nutrients for the endocrine system are high-quality natural fats, which function as precursors to hormones and related substances called prostaglandins. Processed fats, such as refined and hydrogenated vegetable oils and margarine, disrupt hor-mone metabolism and should be avoided. Healthier choices include butter, extra-virgin olive oil, and cold-pressed, unrefined vegetables oils, which are high in essential fatty acids. Flaxseed and evening primrose oil, in particular, have been shown to reduce mood swings associated with PMS and other hormonal changes.

A deficiency of the mineral iodine, an essential nutrient for the thy-roid, can also produce symptoms of depression. Fish and sea vegetables, especially kelp, are good sources of iodine. Cayce often recommended powdered kelp as a substitute for common table salt. The readings also suggest that *Atomidine*, an aqueous solution of iodine from iodine trichloride, is a well-tolerated iodine supplement that can be used for purification and balancing of the glandular system. Reading 358-2 says: *"This [Atomidine] will not only be a curative property, but a* preventative! *May be used internally and externally as well, and especially for any form of disorder in glands or tissue of body."*

The endocrine system responds not only to nutritional therapy, but also to clearing of emotional and energetic blocks. Practitioners of vi-brational medicine, therefore, tend to focus on balancing the chakras, which are focal points in the energy body whose locations correspond to those of the glands in the physical body.

The Cayce readings note that the glands are the locations where the spiritual energies of the soul connect with the body. According to the readings, the glands are influenced by emotions, both positive and negative, thus building or undermining mental and physical health.

Several studies have shown that angry, domineering people are at higher risk of heart disease and high blood pressure. Feelings of anger and depression have been shown to suppress the immune system. Edgar Cayce said, *"Anger may upset the body and cause a great deal of disturbance, to others as well as to self. Be angry but sin not. You will learn it only in patience and in self-possession."* (3621-1) It is important to find ways of dealing with our emotions safely so that they do not cause destruction, to ourselves and others.

The impact that emotions can have on glandular health is demonstrated in a story taken from my file of personal recollections: The thyroid is often associated with the throat chakra, which is related to the energy of personal will and self-expression. In the prime of her life, my mother found herself in extremely stifling circumstances which made it difficult for her to determine the course of her life for many years. She had no opportunity to express her feelings and her creativity freely. She internalized, probably with resentment, all that should have been verbalized and expressed. She developed hyperthyroidism and a massive goiter which, unlike most goiters, could not be seen externally because it had grown toward the inside of her throat. The surgeon who ultimately removed the goiter was awed by its huge size and later apologized for not having taken her complaints of breathlessness seriously much sooner.

As this example suggests, internalizing anger and resentment over long periods of time can result in serious illness. It is important, therefore, that we learn to express our feelings and deal with unresolved issues in a positive, constructive way. In *You Can Heal Your Life*, author Louise Hay says that " . . . thyroid problems are frustrated creativity— not being able to do what you want to do." She recommends an affirmation to help overcome problems related to thyroid conditions: "I move beyond old limitations and now allow myself to express freely and creatively." Consistent use of this affirmation can help transform the emotional and mental energy patterns which trap us in self-limiting, stifling environments and situations.

We can learn from the above that when spiritual self-expression is stifled, the glands react in a way that is physically measurable. To further the expression of the spirit, we can strengthen the chakra connections between the soul and the body through a healthy lifestyle and diet, and especially through meditation and prayer. These disciplines, and the practice of holding a positive attitude, can help us to use our minds in a constructive way—to heal, not hurt, ourselves and others.

Treating Depression Holistically

Depression is the most common behavioral disorder in the world. The number of clinically depressed patients is growing steadily—in 1995, the World Health Organization estimated that there were 100 million worldwide, in 2002, the figure is 120 million. North American statistics indicate that one of three individuals is likely to experience depression during his or her lifetime. Depression costs the U.S. $44 billion per year in lost work productivity.

Clinical depression is different from the occasional sadness, apathy, and dejection most of us feel from time to time, usually in response to a broken relationship, the death of a loved one, or the loss of a job. Fortunately, such feelings dissipate with time or when circumstances change, but clinical depression is much more prolonged and can be profoundly debilitating.

Depression typically manifests itself in chronically low self-esteem and a negative view toward self, others, and life in general. There is often a sense of hopelessness, a lack of interest in other people, the future looks bleak, and life seems totally meaningless. Fatigue, insomnia, lethargy, and the inability to make decisions are some of the symptoms experienced by depressed patients.

The orthodox medical approach is that depression is a disease "of the mind" that is only treatable with antidepressant drugs that alter brain chemistry, as well as with analytical psychotherapy and controversial electroshock treatments. The physical aspect of depression is often ignored or underemphasized. The Cayce readings, however, point out that physical factors are just as important as mental considerations when it comes to the treatment of depression. Mind, body, and spirit cannot be separated from each other. In the readings, one of the major contributing causes of depression is seen as an accumulation of toxic waste materials in the body, due to faulty eliminations which cause the reabsorption of poisons into the bloodstream. Endocrine imbalances are also involved, notably dysfunction of the adrenals, thyroid, and pineal glands. It is fascinating to see research in the third millennium substantiating Cayce's hypothesis. A study reported in the August 2001 issue of the journal *Gut* suggests that women with chronic constipation are more likely to be anxious or depressed than those who don't have bowel problems. Also in 2001, research done at the University of Oxford's Institute of Health Sciences in England showed that patients with ulcerative colitis are considerably more likely to suffer from depression than those who don't have this bowel disease. Both these studies directly confirm the "faulty eliminations" theory in the Cayce readings.

The psychological dimensions of depression are also addressed in the Cayce readings. "Mind is the builder," and therefore patterns of long-held negative attitudes and self-condemnation often manifest as contributing factors. A person's failure to establish a spiritual ideal, and loss of purpose and meaning in life, are also said to play a role in the development of depression.

The holistic treatment suggested in the Cayce readings includes physical detoxification—purifying the system by drinking lots of water and eating natural foods that assist in the process, along with colonic irrigation, massage, spinal manipulation, and castor oil packs. In the Food and Mood section, we have seen how certain nutritional therapies can remedy mental illness, including depression. The readings also recommend physical exercise, especially exercising outdoors in natural sunlight. In chapter 6, we discussed the importance of sunlight for mental and physical health. Treatment with the radial appliance or the wet cell battery (see chapter 6) was also suggested. Prayer, meditation, reading the Bible (especially Deuteronomy 30 and John 14–17), and setting and working with a spiritual ideal were also recommended.

The above therapies are most successful when combined with a program of holistic psychotherapy, which offers a supportive, noninvasive way of successfully dealing with depression and other psychological imbalances. Holistic approaches to psychotherapy help individuals get in touch with the underlying causes of their depression and tap into an inner source of strength from which they are able to redefine their values and consciously establish new, self-sustaining response patterns to life's challenges.

The feelings of despair and helplessness associated with depression are often triggered when an individual, over extended periods of time, has tried to conform to standards which are at variance with their own inner values. In today's achievement-oriented society, individuals tend to be valued in terms of how much they accomplish, so it is not uncommon for someone to view their own worth merely as a reflection of the net-worth figure that their accountant writes on their personal balance sheet.

Often from an early age, children learn that they are not valued for who they are inside but for what they do and accomplish, be it in school or in competition with peers. With parents and teachers as role models, small children develop a critical, judgmental inner voice, which sets the stage for an unconscious pattern of responding to even mildly challenging situations with negative messages such as: "You'll never make it!" or "You're not good enough." Repeatedly played throughout the young person's development into adulthood, such messages are "recorded" into the realm of the subconscious, and tend to trap the individual in the belief that something is wrong with them. To compensate for this perceived inadequacy, they push themselves into over-achievement, getting caught in a desperate pursuit of things "out there" at the expense of other aspects of themselves.

Holistic psychotherapy works with the person to transform this "inner critic" into a voice of support. The individual is encouraged to talk freely about their depression, and to allow feelings and visual impressions to surface which often provide a key for accessing the core issue of their condition. But the strictly intellectual discovery of what troubles the person is not enough, and reexperiencing suppressed trauma without also moving beyond the feelings of fear and pain will only perpetuate the associated sense of helplessness. An important aspect of holistic psychotherapy is the transformational stage, which helps the person to move beyond these feelings into the center of their being, where they are able to feel a strong sense of peace and empowerment.

In order to reach this stage, individuals in therapy are often encouraged to involve different aspects of their being in a "parts play." Aspects which are overemphasized, such as the "accomplisher" in the case of someone who is an overachiever, are brought into balance and peaceful coexistence with other suppressed parts, such as the playful, creative part, which is freed and allowed to express itself with equal force. At this stage, people often discover that the "depressed" part of themselves is not a horrible, shameful thing but just another aspect of themselves demanding attention. Once the overactive and the depressed parts are blended and harmonized, a new oneness is created that encompasses both. The individual no longer feels that there is a conflict between "doing" and "being," but the doing now arises naturally out of their being. Their doing then is in tune with who they really are—they are no longer trying to conform to standards which are not their own.

The suggestions from the Cayce readings to establish a spiritual ideal and work on discovering one's purpose in life are very helpful in aligning life goals and soul purpose. For additional information on this subject, the interested reader is referred to an excellent book, *Soul Purpose*, by Mark A. Thurston, Ph.D. The A.R.E. also sponsors frequent seminars and workshops on *Discovering Your Soul's Purpose* and *Finding Your Mission in Life*.

Having a spiritual ideal and knowing one's soul purpose are important tools in living a life of integrity, as they help to shed light on the ways in which we can reclaim our innate talents as divine gifts to be used for a divine purpose. These tools can help us to move out of a depressed state of being and become happy, healthy, fulfilled, and whole human beings.

The Holistic Treatment of Alcohol Addiction

Alcoholism has a devastating effect on the lives of millions. Nearly one in thirteen adults in the U.S. has a drinking problem, and countless others—family, friends, and co-workers—suffer stress as a result of the alcoholic's addictive behavior. According to substance abuse experts, there was a steep increase in the number of Americans seeking treatment for drug and alcohol abuse during the months following the September 11 attacks on the U.S.

What causes alcohol dependence? Unfortunately, the myth that alcoholism is a mental illness still prevails, and it is commonly believed that alcoholics lack either willpower or strength of character, or have other psychological problems which prevent them from giving up heavy drinking. There is no doubt that an underlying destructive emotional or mental thought pattern is involved in this serious illness. But even though it is generally understood that malnutrition often results from the long-term consumption of alcohol, it is seldom recognized that it is the nutritional deficiencies themselves which severely aggravate and perpetuate alcohol cravings and are directly responsible for the irrational, aggressive, and often violent, behavior of those afflicted with this illness.

Most current treatment and detoxification methods continue to emphasize psychological counseling and rehabilitation, aimed at correcting the underlying emotional and sociological imbalances believed to have triggered the addiction. Nutritional factors are considered secondary and complementary at best. No wonder so few individuals have long-term success in kicking alcohol addiction. Nutritional deficiencies are not eliminated through psychological counseling alone!

Research has shown that deficiencies in important nutrients, such as B-complex vitamins and zinc, lead to increased alcohol cravings and consumption. It has also been demonstrated that an overall improvement in nutritional status through diet and supplements can both reduce alcohol cravings and lessen withdrawal symptoms.

Chronic alcohol abuse is both cause and symptom of nutritional deficiencies. Because it interferes with the absorption of nutrients, alcohol inhibits access to vital amino acids, vitamins, minerals, enzymes, and hormones, thus catapulting the body into a state of malnutrition. By continually triggering insulin reactions from the pancreas, heavy alcohol use contributes to hypoglycemia (low blood sugar), which in turn increases cravings. The pancreas becomes exhausted and unable to produce sufficient digestive enzymes, thus impairing digestion and assimilation.

There is even a nutritional and biochemical connection between chronic alcohol abuse and depression, which so often accompanies this illness. Caught in a roller-coaster ride of biochemical ups and downs, the alcohol addict is unable to gain control over physical cravings, leading to ever deeper feelings of despair, guilt, and hopelessness.

A sound nutrition plan which supplies all necessary nutrients in optimal amounts can help to bring the body back into balance, detoxify the system, and prevent a recurrence of cravings. Here are some of the most important nutrients to consider:

Vitamin B Complex.   Heavy alcohol consumption depletes B vitamins, which are essential for proper brain and nervous system function. Depression, confusion, memory loss, and insomnia, are some of the symptoms of vitamin B deficiency which are also associated with alcoholism. Supplementation with B complex reduces cravings and restores the health of the nervous system. Choline and inositol, which are cofactors in the function of B vitamins, are also important for the repair of alcohol–induced liver damage. (Therapeutic dosage: 150 to 200 mg/day)

Vitamin A.   Progressive alcoholic liver disease can result in failure of the liver to store vitamin A. Supplementation is therefore important to prevent deficiencies of this important nutrient. It also helps to alleviate potential liver dysfunction. (Therapeutic dosage: 10,000 to 25,000 IU/day)

Vitamin C.   Vitamin C is a powerful detoxifier. Supplementation with this vitamin has been shown to reverse addictive states and to reduce the effects of alcohol toxicity. For best results, use a buffered (with calcium) form of vitamin C, which is less acidic in the body. The addition of bioflavonoids increases the effectiveness and bioavailability of vitamin C. (Therapeutic dosage: 3,000 to 6,000 mg/day)

Calcium/Magnesium.   Heavy ingestion of alcohol severely increases calcium and magnesium output, producing symptoms such as muscle tremors and cramps, changes in heart rhythm, irritability, insomnia, slow reflexes, and emotional instability. Chronic alcohol use can lead to reduced bone mass and osteomalacia, a softening of the bones in adults. Impaired liver function in alcoholics results in an inability of the liver to hydroxylate vitamin D, which further aggravates a calcium deficiency. Convulsive seizures and delirium result from seriously depleted magnesium levels.

When choosing a supplement, look for a readily assimilable form of calcium, such as hydroxyapatite, citrate, or phosphate, in a 2:1 ratio with magnesium. (Therapeutic dosage: 1,000 to 1,400 mg [calcium]/day)

Zinc. Zinc is a cofactor for alcohol dehydrogenase, which works in the liver to detoxify alcohol. Chronic alcohol consumption is associated with zinc deficiency. Supplementation with this important mineral can lessen withdrawal symptoms and help to prevent seizures and brain dysfunction. Normalizing zinc levels also reduces alcohol cravings. (Therapeutic dosage: 50 to 80 mg/day)

Essential Fatty Acids (EFAs). Excessive alcohol intake severely disrupts EFA metabolism by blocking the conversion of linoleic acid to gamma-linolenic acid (GLA), required for the formation of prostaglandin E1, an important factor in brain metabolism. An alcohol-induced deficiency can be prevented or eliminated by supplementing the diet with oil of evening primrose or borage oil, two of only a few known sources of dietary GLA. Supplementation helps to diminish alcohol withdrawal symptoms and to improve liver function. (Therapeutic dosage: 3,000 mg/day)

Amino Acids. Amino acids are the building blocks of protein which the body extracts from food sources. Amino acids are also required for the production of specific brain chemicals (neurotransmitters) which determine moods and emotions. In alcoholics, amino acid metabolism is often impaired and conversion to neurotransmitters is disrupted, resulting in mental confusion, aggressive behavior, and depression. Supplementation has been shown to reduce alcohol intoxication, balance moods, and diminish the desire for alcohol. Of special importance are L-cysteine and L-glycine. (Therapeutic dosage: 1,500 mg/day)

Other nutrients which play a role in controlling metabolic damage from excessive alcohol consumption include vitamin E, chromium, iron, phosphorus, and selenium. Heavy alcohol use can also contribute to food allergies, thyroid disorders, and Candida in the intestinal tract. As well, each of these conditions can aggravate cravings for alcohol. A naturopathic physician or holistic medical health professional can help to determine the best nutrition plan and supplementation program so that specific deficiencies are properly addressed.

The Cayce readings acknowledge the important role that physical influences play in alcohol addiction. Spinal manipulation was sometimes recommended, as was treatment with the wet cell battery. In reading 1439-1, a thirty–eight–year–old man, who asked if he was correct in his belief that he successfully conquered the addiction, was told:

> *This may not be accomplished until there is removed* physically *those pressures that cause the inability of the system, between the nervous forces of the body, to prevent the possession of the appetites seeking desire by influences without as well as gratification within.*

The young man was not satisfied with this explanation and continued to question the sleeping Cayce: *"Other than when distorted by alcohol, is there any reason to believe the mind is in any way sick? I would like to have a concrete analysis to substantiate your opinion."* He received the following response:

> *This has been given as to how and why. For the effect upon the organs of the system makes for an* illness *in the physical body, finding expression in the mental outside of self and in the gratifying of appetites within self.*
>
> *So the mental is not ill but misdirected by influences from pressures within and influences from without.*
>
> *With the removal of these pressures, the toning and tuning of the system for a more normal activity, and with the mental self made more* constructive *in its reactions, we should find a change that would make for a concrete example of the whole effect of the influences of constructive thought as applied in the mental self.*

This reading emphasizes the correction of both physical and mental aspects in healing the young man's alcohol dependency, who then asked another question of Cayce: *"In connection with the proper care of mind and body, is there any particular food recommended?"* Cayce replied:

> *Only those that are of a correct balance in the acidity and alkalinity of the system. Do not use too great a quantity of starches that de-*

mand those influences to produce an overabundance of alcoholic re-
action.   *1439-1*

Cayce's nutritional recommendations are not as complex and elaborate as those outlined above. But I have quoted from this reading to
demonstrate that the information provided in the Cayce readings leaves
no doubt that physical care is often required in the treatment of substance abuse, just as it is necessary in the treatment of depression. In at
least one reading for a victim of alcoholism, Cayce recommended a
combination of eucalyptol, rectified oil of turpentine, benzosol, and
codeine to be administered while under a physician's care. This remedy
was intended to produce a reaction within the patient so that he would
become sick when taking alcohol. This is still the principle behind some
of the medications given to alcoholics today.

Another reading for an alcoholic, one which recommended treatment with the wet cell battery using a combination of chloride of gold
and bromide of soda, stressed the uniqueness of each case of addiction,
pointing out that not all addictions are caused by physical factors. Cayce
was asked: *"In alcoholic cases, can a general outline of treatment be given?"* His
reply:

No. Each individual has its own individual problems. Not all are
physical. *Hence there are those that are of the sympathetic nature,*
or where there has been the possession by the very activity of same;
but gold will destroy desire in any of them!   *606-1*

In a follow-up reading for the thirty-eight-year-old alcohol addict
who had asked if his mind was ill in any other way, Cayce was asked:
"Can those assisting do anything to prevent the body from indulging in stimulants?"
He replied:

They can pray like the devil!
And this is not a blasphemous statement, as it may appear—to
some. For if there is any busier body, with those influences that have
to do with the spirit of indulgence of any nature, than that ye call
satan or the devil, who is it?

Then it behooves those who have the interest of such a body at heart to not only pray for him but with him; and in just as earnest, just as sincere, just as continuous a manner as the spirit of any indulgence works upon those who have become subject to such influences either through physical, mental or material conditions!

For the power of prayer is not met even by satan or the devil himself.

Hence with that attitude of being as persistent as the desire for indulgence, or as persistent as the devil, ye will find ye will bring a strength. But if ye do so doubting, ye are already half lost.

For the desires of the body are to do right! *Then aid those desires in the right direction; for the power of right exceeds—ever and always.*

Do that, then.

*Like the devil himself—*pray!   1439-2

Mind as Healer

The assertion that "spirit is life, *mind is the builder*, physical is the result" is a recurrent theme in the Cayce readings. It is the mind that molds spiritual energy into physical manifestation, creating health or illness. Attitudes that are habitually (and often unconsciously) held in the mind influence the way in which this molding process unfolds. The word *attitude* can be traced back to its Latin root, the verb *aptare*, meaning to "put on." An attitude is like a filter that we put on the mind, and which colors our perception according to the shade we have chosen. As such, we might see the world optimistically, through rose–colored glasses, so to speak, or negatively, through a dark shade. And just as we sometimes forget that we are wearing glasses of a certain shade, we might forget that the filter we have put on our mind is, in fact, removable and can be replaced whenever we choose to do so.

The Cayce readings say *"a great many of the angles or attitudes in the physical forces of the body are brought about by the mental attitude that is held—and through same make for those building influences in the body."* (270–34) Reading 4021–1 depicts in no uncertain terms in what way such attitudes can manifest as illness in the body: *"To be sure, attitudes oft influence the physical conditions of the body. No one can hate his neighbor and not have stomach or liver trouble. No one can be jealous and allow the anger of same and not have upset digestion or heart disorder."* The readings emphasize the importance of an optimistic, constructive, and positively expectant attitude: *"Keep optimistic and prayerful, and with a song on the lips often, if you want the body to be cheerful!"* (23–11) and *"Keep the mental attitude in a constructive manner. Know within self that the physical elements may be builded; that the Mind is the Builder; that the manner in which the spiritual influences and forces may act upon the system builds that which is held in the deeper mental force. Keep it, then,* constructive! *Do not think negatively."* (1074–1)

In the year 2000, researchers at the prestigious Mayo Clinic reported that they had found optimists to live longer, healthier, and more successful lives than pessimists. Since then, several additional studies have corroborated these findings. A study reported in the March 23, 2001, issue of *Psychosomatic Medicine* once again confirmed the mind–body connection by showing that an optimistic, hopeful attitude may help to reduce the risk of stroke in the elderly. Even among patients who have suffered a stroke, those who maintain an optimistic, hopeful outlook considerably improve their chances for survival, according to a report in the July 2001 issue of *Stroke: Journal of the American Heart Association.* Similarly, research has shown that an optimistic attitude could act as a protective mechanism against heart disease and that patient expectations had a direct influence on recovery. In other words, when patients expected to get better, they did.

What does this suggest about how we should view illness, including chronic degenerative disease? As an affliction that we are required to carry with us for the rest of our lives and that will only get worse as we age? Or as a remedial process that can teach us where we have gone wrong and that, with the correct application of appropriate remedial measures and a positive mental outlook, will no longer be in effect once the healing is accomplished? What about saying, day in and day out, that "we *have*" a disease? Do we really want to go around proclaiming ownership of an illness and continuously affirming, to ourselves and to others, that we are its victims? Do we want to give mental and verbal affirmation to the belief that certain diseases are "incurable"? If we believe and affirm that a particular disease will continuously weaken us and ultimately get the better of us and kill us, we can be sure that we are writing the script of a self-fulfilling prophecy. Every doctor's records are full of unexplained spontaneous remissions and miraculous recoveries, but we need to mentally claim them as our own, rather than making a claim for the illness. Cayce reading 2948-1 boldly recommends: "Do *keep sweet. Keep that attitude of expectancy. Do keep the attitude of hope. And* know *that there is healing in the power and might of the love of God.*"

Jay D. Allen, an inspirational speaker and seminar leader, writes in his book *Humans in Training: An Owner's Manual* about his challenge of being diagnosed with a brain tumor at the age of eighteen and receiving a prediction from doctors that he had only fifteen months to live. Not giving power to the diagnosis, he responded by turning within through intense study, meditation, and contemplation of spiritual teachings. When he published his book fifteen years later, doctors could not explain why he was still alive. Today, Jay is teaching others about the powers of the mind, and how to use them to overcome adverse circumstances, including ill health. He writes in *Humans In Training*: "All the great teachers and masters have warned us to be careful of how and what we think because thought is energy—an actual living thing. We create the world with our thoughts . . . everything exists first on the plane of thought and eventually spirals down to the physical plane."

We can use our minds to create health, illness, even death. It's just a matter of expectation, faith, and attitude. A study published in the *British Medical Journal* for December 22/29, 2001, showed that certain culturally held superstitious beliefs have a measurable effect on mortality. According to the study, Chinese and Japanese Americans with heart disease appear to be at greater risk of dying of a heart attack on the fourth day of any given month. The number four is considered to be an "unlucky" number in China and Japan because the word "four" sounds very similar to the word "death" in both the Chinese and Japanese languages.

The idea that a change of mind can bring about different physical conditions is also the underlying principle in hypnosis and hypnotherapy. In the Introduction, we discussed the remarkable story of how Edgar Cayce was cured of aphonia—the loss of his voice—in an experiment involving hypnosis. Recent research has shown that hypnotherapy is effective in reducing pain and anxiety during surgery, that it helps to improve irritable bowel syndrome, and that it may be helpful as an adjunct in asthma therapy. Self–hypnosis has been shown to help those who respond to certain environmental triggers with pathological symptoms such as asthma attacks, to keep such reactions under control. Research done at Beth Israel Deaconess Medical Center in Boston, Massachusetts, even showed that the use of hypnosis in the operating room could cut the costs of some medical procedures in half by reducing pain and stress on the patient, and lessening the need for medication after the surgery.

The Cayce readings recommended hypnosis in some cases, while advising against it in others, favoring instead the use of suggestive therapy, prayer, and meditation. A fifty–five–year–old woman suffering from Parkinson's disease, for instance, asked in reading 3450–1: *"Would hypnosis help the body conditions? If so, please give name and address of reliable hypnotist in or near Boston."* Cayce replied: *"Not as we find indicated here. Spirituality is the most help. Deep meditation, prayer, will be the most helpful."*

Reading 146–3, given for a deaf–mute thirteen–year–old boy with epilepsy, features the following dialogue:

(Q) Could hypnotism be used in his case?
(A) It might be used, but be mindful *of who would use same!*
(Q) Would auto-suggestion be helpful?
(A) Most beneficial. This can be given best by [the] mother.

Therapy by making suggestion to the patient, especially at the time that he or she is drifting off to sleep, was often recommended in the readings, particularly for children and adolescents.

When asked in reading 3744–3 to explain the difference in suggestion to the subconscious mind and the conscious mind, Edgar Cayce answered:

Suggestion to the conscious mind only brings to the mental plane those forces that are of the same character and the conscious is the suggestion in action. In that of suggestion to the subconscious mind, it gives its reflection or reaction from the universal forces or mind or superconscious forces. By the suggestion just as given may be wavered by the forces that are brought to bear on the subconscious to reach the conscious mind, just as we have in a purely mechanical form. Any object, or wood especially, projected into water, appears bent; just so with the reflection from suggestions to the subconscious to reach the conscious or mental forces appear bent in their action, or in the manifestation of their action, to the physical or conscious forces of individuals.

The readings also suggest visualization as a means of bringing healing to the body, saying *"The body should see self as it desires itself to be!"* (275–17) and *"If the body will aid self in those applications as may be made for same, see self—in the period when the body enters into the quiet—healed as it, the body, would be healed."* (326–1)

Visualization can be seen as a way of making self–suggestions to the mind—sending instructions to the mind, which is the builder, as given in reading 5642–5: " . . . *the* mental *is the Builder. See self with the added forces necessary for the corrections, as* well and strong, *and revibrating to the new flow of blood and energy as is being created in the system by the proper vibrations being set up in the physical body, and we will find the body will respond and build that image so held before its inner self."* Visualization as an adjunct to therapy is used in many alternative and complementary cancer recovery programs. Patients visualize tumors dissolving and cancerous tissue being destroyed and transformed into healthy cells. The Cayce readings energetically and positively affirm that it is possible through visualization to heal self and build a healthy body: *"Let nature and the mind itself see self improving.* Hold *the idea, the ideal. That as desired may be builded."* (3838–1)

Prayer and Meditation.   Research has shown that having an active religious or spiritual life, good friends, an effective support network, laughter, and a forgiving attitude toward others can all boost our health and promote healing. All these, in various ways, engage our spiritual selves and bring spiritual energies into our day–to–day activities and interactions with others. The readings assert: " . . . *know that it is the activating of the spiritual forces within the body that brings, that must bring, healing."* (2703–1) Nothing quickens the spiritual forces within more than prayer—direct communication with God. The Bible says, *"Pray for one another, so that you may be healed."* (James 5:16) We have Jesus' assurance that our prayers are answered by God: *"Ask, and it shall be given you; seek, and ye shall find; knock, and it shall be opened unto you: for every one that asketh receiveth; and he that seeketh findeth; and to him that knocketh it shall be opened."* (Matt. 7:7–8 KJV)

In her inspiring book *Rediscovering Your Authentic Self*, which is based on the principles of *A Course in Miracles*, Moreah Ragusa Fach writes: "Prayer and meditation are powerful tools to reinstate our true identity to our awareness. Prayer is a way of acknowledging an acceptance of our relationship to our Father. Prayer and meditation bring feelings of empowerment, comfort, and peace to many people. This is true primarily for one reason, and that is that when we pray, we communicate with our Creator and once again establish our oneness. Both scientists and Western medical professionals have studied the power of prayer and its effects on those who are ill. It has been discovered that patients who are being prayed for return to health 60 percent quicker than those who are not prayed for. This is really not so mysterious when we understand that mind is shared. As one of us accepts our totality, all of us receive the benefits. Ultimately, healing is increased because identity is being shared and acknowledged."

The Cayce readings offer an undeniably strong message regarding the effectiveness of prayer in healing: *"Then, more may be accomplished in prayer than in medication."* (3289-1) A report published in the October 25, 1999, issue of the *Archives of Internal Medicine* talks about a double-blind study conducted with hospitalized heart patients. One group of heart patients were prayed for daily for four weeks by a fifteen-member team of self-identified, practicing Christians. At the end of the experiment, the patients who had been prayed for had significantly fewer complications than those who had not been prayed for as part of this study. Neither the doctors nor the patients knew who was on the list of those being prayed for. The results of this study confirm the findings of earlier research done in San Francisco in 1988. Other recent experiments with prayer have shown that prayer boosts the success of in vitro fertilization and that it can directly influence the growth or suppression of bacteria in a culture.

It has also been demonstrated that prayer, thought, and sound have a measurable effect on the structure and shape of water molecules. This is documented in Dr. Masaru Emoto's fascinating book *Messages from Water*. In the studies described by Dr. Emoto, water molecules responded to labels pasted on water bottles with the same speed as to the effect of long-distance prayer aimed at the water. The messages written on the labels were either loving or hateful, and the water crystals correspondingly would take on highly harmonious and beautiful or extremely ugly shapes, depending on the message or the prayer. When we consider the fact that the human body consists of 70 percent water, it becomes easy to understand how we can influence our own and others' bodies with thought and prayer.

Another study, which showed that the rhythmic chanting used by individuals saying the rosary prayer, as well as when performing yoga mantras, has a calming effect on the heart, demonstrates that prayer is nondenominational. Both the recitation of the rosary and the yoga mantra synchronized heart rhythms in an identical pattern, reducing the respiratory rate to a very healthy six breaths per minute.

Astonishing results were also seen in studies involving meditation, a practice highly recommended by Edgar Cayce. Reading 1223–7 says, *"Have regular periods of rest, and use these as the periods of meditation; and we will find all of the activities, physical, mental and spiritual, will be much better coordinated . . . "* Meditation has been shown to provide short-term relief from asthma attacks, and to lower blood pressure. One study reported in the March 2000 issue of *Stroke: Journal of the American Heart Association*, showed that signs of atherosclerosis—the accumulation of fatty plaque material on artery walls—diminished in test subjects who were meditating on a regular basis.

The Cayce readings recommend prayer and meditation as a tool for healing both self and others, saying that as healing is received for self, it must be passed on to others for it to be of lasting value. Reading 281–18 says: *"Healing others is healing self. For, to give out that which aids others in reaching that which creates the perfect vibration of life in their physical selves, through the mental attitudes and aptitudes of the body, brings to self better understanding."* Research reported in the September 28, 2001, issue of the *Journal of the American Psychoanalytic Association* focused on altruism, particularly in connection with incidents of self-sacrifice that were made public following the terrorist attacks on the World Trade Center and the Pentagon. The researchers concluded that while altruism is a complex human characteristic, it has more than basic instinctual roots, giving people a reason to feel good about themselves, by doing something that helps others and makes them feel better. Not being able to help when tragedy strikes, not being able "to do something," results in frustration.

We are all part of the human family, and we are "wired" to want to support each other. Indeed, it makes sense to do so. Quantum physics has discovered that all of creation is connected in a single field of energy. Every human in this world is linked in consciousness with every other human and everything in existence. Every personal and collective thought, every emotion, every deed, directly and immediately affects this energy field. Ultimately, our thoughts and actions are mirrored back to us in our relationships, our surroundings, and globally in world events. The microcosm reflected in the macrocosm—as within, so without. Cayce reading 1246-2 states: " . . . *if ye would know joy, give joy* . . . "

As we ask for and receive healing for our bodies and our minds, may our prayers be that we may become channels of healing for others—our brothers and sisters with whom we share this magical, mystical journey through time and space on planet earth.

Note: The A.R.E. Prayer Services department continues a tradition begun by the original Glad Helpers Prayer Group started by Edgar Cayce back in 1931. Each month approximately 4,500 individuals around the world receive the International Prayer List. These individuals have generously agreed to meditate daily and pray for others on the prayer list. To place yourself or others on the prayer list, contact: A.R.E. Prayer Services, 215 67th Street, Virginia Beach, VA 23451-2061.

Bibliography

An Edgar Cayce Home Medicine Guide
A.R.E. Press, Virginia Beach, VA, 1982

Ancient Indian Massage
by Harish Johari
Munshiram Manoharlal Publishers Pvt. Ltd., New Delhi, 1984

A Time to Heal: How to Reap the Benefits of Holistic Health
by Daniel Redwood, D.C.
A.R.E. Press, Virginia Beach, VA, 1993

Auras
by Edgar Cayce
A.R.E. Press, Virginia Beach, VA, 1994

Ayurvedic Healing
by Dr. David Frawley, O.M.D.
Motilal Banarsidass Publishers Pvt. Ltd., Delhi, India, 1994

Confessions of a Medical Heretic
by Robert S. Mendelsohn, M.D.
Warner Books, Inc., New York, NY, 1979

Dian Dincin Buchman's Herbal Medicine: The Natural Way to Get Well and Stay Well
Gramercy Publishing Company, NY, 1980

Heal Arthritis: Physically—Mentally—Spiritually
by William A. McGarey, M.D.
A.R.E. Press, Virginia Beach, VA, 1998

Healing Psoriasis: The Natural Alternative
by Dr. John O.A. Pagano
The Pagano Organization, Inc., Englewood Cliffs, NJ, 1991

Healing Through Meditation and Prayer
by Meredith Ann Puryear
A.R.E. Press, Virginia Beach, VA, 1999

Humans in Training: An Owner's Manual
 by Jay D. Allen
 HIT Publishing, Newmarket, ON, Canada, 2003

Light: Medicine of the Future
 by Jacob Liberman, O.D., Ph.D.
 Bear & Company Publishing, Santa Fe, NM, 1991

Light, Radiation & You
 by John N. Ott
 Devin-Adair, Greenwich, CT, 1990

Messages from Water
 by Masaru Emoto
 Koha, Japan, 2002

Music as the Bridge
 by Shirley Rabb Winston
 A.R.E. Press, Virginia Beach, VA, 1972

Nature Doctors: Pioneers in Naturopathic Medicine
 by Friedhelm Kirchfeld & Wade Boyle
 Medicina Biologica, Portland, OR, 1994

Nourishing the Body Temple
 by Simone Gabbay
 A.R.E. Press, Virginia Beach, VA, 1999

Nourishing Traditions
 by Sally Fallon, with Pat Connolly and Mary G. Enig, Ph.D.
 ProMotion Publishing, San Diego, CA, 1995

Planetary Herbology: An Integration of Western Herbs into the Traditional Chinese and Ayurvedic Systems
 by Michael Tierra, C.A., N.D.
 Lotus Press, Santa FE, NM, 1988

Rediscovering Your Authentic Self
 by Moreah Ragusa Fach

Angels Answers Inc., Okotoks, AB, Canada, 2002

Self-Healing: My Life and Vision
by Meir Schneider
Arkana, Viking Penguin Inc., New York, NY, 1989

Seven Weeks to Sobriety: The Proven Program to Fight Alcoholism Through Nutrition
by Joan Mathews Larson, Ph.D.
Random House, Toronto, Canada, 1992

Soul Purpose: Discovering and Fulfilling Your Destiny
by Mark A. Thurston, Ph.D.
St. Martin's Press, New York, NY, 1997

Spiritual Nutrition and the Rainbow Diet
by Gabriel Cousins, M.D.
Cassandra Press, SanRafael, CA, 1986

The Complete Book of Juicing
by Michael T. Murray, N.D.
Prima Publishing, Rocklin, CA, 1992

The Complete Edgar Cayce Readings for Windows (CD-ROM)
A.R.E. Press, Virginia Beach, VA, 1995

The Edgar Cayce Handbook for Health Through Drugless Therapy
by Dr. Harold J. Reilly and Ruth Hagy Brod
A.R.E. Press, Virginia Beach, VA, 1975

The Edgar Cayce Way of Overcoming Multiple Sclerosis: Vibratory Medicine
by Dr. Dudley Delany
Meridian Publications, Hampton, VA, 1999

The Encyclopedia of Essential Oils
by Julia Lawless
Element, Inc., Rockport, MA, 1992

The Fragrant Pharmacy
by Valerie Ann Worwood

Bantam Books, London, UK, 1990

The Handbook of Self-Healing
 by Meir Schneider and Maureen Larkin with Dror Schneider
 by Arkana, Penguin Books, New York, NY, 1994

The Memory of Water: Homeopathy and the Battle of Ideas in the New Science
 by Michel Schiff
 Thorsons, San Francisco, CA, 1995

Messages from Water
 by Masaru Emoto
 Earth Traditions, Idyllwild, CA, 2002

The Miracle of Suggestion
 by Cynthia Pike Ouellette
 Inner Vision Publishing Co., Virginia Beach, VA, 1988

The Natural Family Doctor
 by Dr. Andrew Stanway, MB, MRCP
 with Richard Grossman, Ph.D.
 Simone & Schuster, Inc., New York, NY, 1987

The Nutritional Cost of Prescription Drugs: How to Maintain Good Nutrition while Using Prescription Drugs
 by Ross Pelton, R.Ph., and James B. LaValle, R.Ph.
 Morton Publishing Company, Englewood, CO, 2000

The Oil That Heals: A Physician's Successes with Castor Oil Treatments
 by William A. McGarey, M.D.,
 A.R.E. Press, Virginia Beach, VA, 1995

The Scientific Validation of Herbal Medicine
 by Daniel B. Mowrey, Ph.D.
 Keats Publishing, New Canaan, Conn., 1986

The Secret Music of the Soul
 by Patrick Bernhardt
 Imagine Records & Publishing, St-Sauveur, Quebec, Canada, 1991

Why We Live after Death
    by Dr. Richard Steinpach
    Grail Foundation Press
    Gambier, Ohio, 1996

You Can Heal Your Life
    by Louise L. Hay
    Hay House Inc., Santa Monica, CA, 1988

Your Body's Many Cries for Water: You Are Not Sick, You Are Thirsty
    by Fereydoon Batmanghelidj
    Global Health Solutions, July 1997

Index

Glands 52, 79, 102, 119, 148, 149, 150, 152
Glyco–Thymoline 104, 111

H

Headaches xiii, 2, 3, 5, 7, 28, 53, 72, 75, 89,
    112, 113, 114, 120, 130
Herbs xv, 4, 5, 48, 52, 71, 94, 96, 97, 98, 100,
    102, 103, 104, 108, 111, 114, 115
Homeopathy 3, 4, 108, 133, 134, 135
Hydrotherapy xvi, 3, 46, 49, 71, 73, 76, 108
Hypoglycemia 144, 155

I

Immune system 8, 20, 28, 31, 40, 42, 58,
    59, 61, 123, 127, 134, 150
Ipsab 104, 114

J

Jerusalem artichoke 45, 46, 144

L

Lavender 94, 109, 110, 112, 114, 118, 120,
    121, 122, 143
Lymph system 58, 59, 60

M

Massage xv, xvi, xvii, 2, 3, 4, 49, 51, 53, 54,
    56, 57, 58, 59, 60, 62, 63, 64, 65, 67, 74,
    75, 76, 77, 104, 110, 113, 114, 118, 121,
    122, 152
Memory 7, 66, 88, 90, 130, 135, 140, 141,
    142, 145, 146, 147, 148, 156
Mental disorders 139, 140
Meridian Institute xviii
Migraines 2, 113, 114
Mind xiii, xv, xvii, xviii, 2, 13, 14, 18, 49,
    69, 78, 90, 116, 117, 120, 123, 130, 133,
    139, 140, 141, 142, 143, 144, 151, 152,
    158, 159, 160, 161, 162, 163, 164, 165,
    167
Multiple sclerosis xiii, xvii, 7, 136, 137
Mummy food 147
Music 124, 130, 131, 132, 133

N

Naturopathy 2, 71, 108

Nervous tension xv, 99, 136

O

Osteopathy xv, 54, 55, 56, 57, 64, 76
Osteoporosis 7, 47, 80, 83
Overweight 12, 35

P

Posture 82, 85
Prayer 14, 50, 68, 116, 117, 118, 133, 151,
    152, 160, 161, 163, 164, 165, 166, 167
Psoriasis xvii, 41, 100, 101, 102, 136

R

Radial Appliance xvii, 136, 137, 138, 152
Rest 58, 77, 86, 88, 92, 129, 142, 144, 166

S

Salt 20, 31, 37, 38, 39, 49, 80, 104, 111, 113,
    114, 149
Schizophrenia 18, 90, 137, 139, 146
Sleep 58, 84, 86, 87, 88, 89, 90, 91, 92, 93,
    94, 95, 101, 112, 128, 132, 134, 143,
    146, 163
Sound therapy 131
Spirit xiii, xv, xvii, 2, 16, 49, 58, 66, 67, 68,
    69, 73, 86, 92, 114, 116, 117, 118, 119,
    123, 124, 125, 130, 131, 137, 143, 147,
    149, 150, 151, 152, 154, 160, 161, 163,
    164, 166
Stress 2, 14, 38, 49, 53, 65, 69, 81, 87, 88, 89,
    90, 111, 113, 130, 131, 138, 142, 143,
    144, 145, 147, 154
Sugar 6, 12, 18, 25, 26, 28, 31, 32, 40, 44, 46,
    70, 95, 105, 108, 134, 144, 145, 147, 148,
    155
Sunshine 33, 81, 82, 125, 126, 129, 144
Supplements 4, 5, 32, 34, 40, 44, 46, 48, 52,
    67, 106, 107, 112, 126, 146, 149, 155

T

Tai Chi 84
Therapeutic Touch 51, 68, 69
Thyroid 28, 36, 38, 49, 149, 150, 152, 157
Touch 50, 51, 58, 68, 118, 120, 125, 152

A.R.E. Press

The A.R.E. Press publishes books, videos, and audiotapes meant to improve the quality of our readers' lives—personally, professionally, and spiritually. We hope our products support your endeavors to realize your career potential, to enhance your relationships, to improve your health, and to encourage you to make the changes necessary to live a loving, joyful, and fulfilling life.

For more information or to receive a free catalog, call:

1–800–723–1112

Or write:

A.R.E. Press
215 67th Street
Virginia Beach, VA 23451–2061

Baar Products

A.R.E.'s Official Worldwide Exclusive Supplier of Edgar Cayce Health Care Products

Baar Products, Inc., is the official worldwide exclusive supplier of Edgar Cayce health care products. Baar offers a collection of natural products and remedies drawn from the work of Edgar Cayce, considered by many to be the father of modern holistic medicine.

For a complete listing of Cayce–related products, call:

1–800–269–2502

Or write:

Baar Products, Inc.
P.O. Box 60
Downingtown, PA 19335 U.S.A.

Customer Service and International: 610–873–4591
Fax: 610–873–7945
Web Site: www.baar.com   E-mail: cayce@baar.com